Acid Reflux

Learn How to Cure Acid Reflux Naturally

(A Complete Cookbook With Low Acid Recipes to Cure and Prevent Gerd)

William Castillo

Published By **John Kembrey**

William Castillo

Acid Reflux: Learn How to Cure Acid Reflux Naturally (A Complete Cookbook With Low Acid Recipes to Cure and Prevent Gerd)

ISBN **978-1-998769-30-8**

No part of this guidebook shall be reproduced in any form without permission in writing from the publisher except in the case of brief quotations embodied in critical articles or reviews.

Legal & Disclaimer

The information contained in this ebook is not designed to replace or take the place of any form of medicine or professional medical advice. The information in this ebook has been provided for educational & entertainment purposes only.

The information contained in this book has been compiled from sources deemed reliable, and it is accurate to the best of the Author's knowledge; however, the Author cannot guarantee its accuracy and validity and cannot be held liable for any errors or omissions. Changes are periodically made to this book. You must consult your doctor or get professional medical advice before using any of the suggested remedies, techniques, or information in this book.

Table Of Contents

Table Of Contents

Chapter 1: What Acid Reflux Gerd Is

Acid Reflux Disease

acid re·flux: heartburn caused by
regurgitation —upward ejection of acid
from the stomach into the esophagus,
causing pain known as heartburn

The reason for acid reflux is by definition heartburn that is caused by regurgitation. upward expulsion of stomach acid into the esophagus. This causes discomfort or pain called heartburn. This is the standard definition.

Acid Reflux Disease

- Gastroesophageal reflux disease (GERD) is a chronic symptom of mucosal damage caused by stomach acid coming up from the stomach into the esophagus.[1]
- GERD is usually caused by changes in the barrier between the stomach and the esophagus, including abnormal relaxation of the lower esophageal sphincter, which normally holds the top of the stomach closed, impaired expulsion of gastric reflux from the esophagus, or a hiatal hernia. These changes may be permanent or temporary.
- Treatment is typically via lifestyle changes and medications such as proton pump inhibitors, H₂ receptor blockers or antacids. Surgery may be an option in those who do not improve. In the Western world between 10 and 20% of the population is affected.

More Info About Acid Reflux

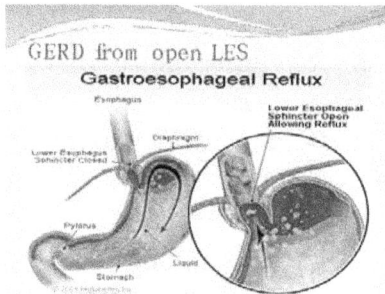

GERD from open LES

Gastroesophageal Reflux

Esophagus

Lower Esophageal Sphincter Open Allowing Reflux

Diaphragm

Lower Esophageal Sphincter Closed

Pylorus

Liquid

Stomach

It's typically a manifestation of damage to the mucosa caused by stomach acid flowing through the stomach in the esophagus. The barrier that separates the stomach and the esophagus, the sphincter is a muscle similar to the one in the

2

urethra or rectum There's a sphincter located in the middle of the esophagus muscles which contracts to prevent acidic foods from coming down. When you consume food, it relaxes and allows food to pass through. When the food is gone, it is believed to tighten up, and prevents signs of acid reflux.

Some people might have hiatal hernias and changes could occur and disappear up to an Sphincter. The treatment can involve a range of aspects, including lifestyle modifications - I'll discuss these, as well as different types of drugs. You're probably familiar with items like simple antacidsand antagonists of H2, receptor blockers proton pump inhibitors and even surgical procedures, generally reserved for patients who are not managed on any of those other medications.

In the case of GERD, it is from Open LES

They claim that GERD is so prevalent that anywhere from 10 to 20 percent of the population are affected by this disease. Here's one small image where it shows the stomach filled with fluids within the diaphragm. The image illustrates a gap between stomach contents or the abdominal contents, and the lung. The lung is situated above the diaphragm. It is the sphincter which restricts food from flowing normally. However, sometimes, as shown in the tiny circle it is apparent that the muscles may not be fully contracted and fluids including stomach acid could be resurfacing and cause irritation, inflammation and burning, which can cause discomfort, and sometimes not but I'll discuss the symptoms in a bit.

The unpleasant symptoms of acid Reflux

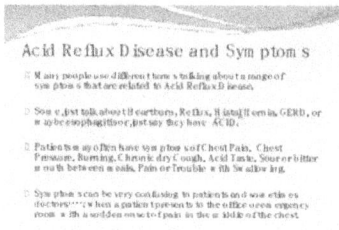

Acid Reflux Disease and Symptoms

- Many people use different terms talking about a range of symptoms that are related to Acid Reflux Disease.

- Some just talk about Heartburn, Reflux, Hiatal Hernia, GERD, or acid or esophagitis or, just say they have ACID.

- Patients may often have symptoms of Chest Pain, Chest Pressure, Burning, Chronic dry Cough, Acid Taste, Sour or bitter mouth between meals, Pain or Trouble with Swallowing.

- Symptoms can be very confusing to patients and sometimes doctors, when a patient presents to the office or an emergency room with a sudden onset of pain in the middle of the chest.

There are many people who are talking about various terms associated with acid reflux. Some declare it's heartburn or simply refer to it as reflux or hiatal hernia. It is a particular kind of

4

condition, when talking about it. Many people refer to it as GERD which is gastro esophageal resuscitation disease. certain people simply say I've got acid. The symptoms of GERD are often severe that may include chest tension, pain, or burning, and many times , there's dry, chronic cough in which tiny bits of acid entering the lungs and causing irritation but they don't notice it happening. Esophageal symptoms might experience an acidic taste or a bitter and sharp taste inside their mouths during meals, and occasionally it may get to the point where they feel pain or difficulties with eating particularly if there's been an extended period of inflammation, or perhaps scarring or tightness.

The issue is that symptoms can be difficult for patients, and sometimes to doctors too when you experience chest pain. This is why you might visit the doctor's office or to the emergency department with discomfort, but you might not be aware, and the doctor may not be able to tell, even for a long time whether there's something major happening or not. So, is this reflux caused by heartburn or acid, or is it actually an attack of the heart? This is obviously a significant distinction.

Chest Pain - Could it be GERD?

Here's a different picture and you're thinking whether the discomfort, is it because of drinking coffee? The first thing to consider is that it's the case that it's not Boresha Coffee, which doesn't cause it but, is he suffering from heartburn or is he suffering from an attack on his heart? This is why I'm here to provide you with a further on this.

What Doctors Test for In an Emergency Room

One of the most common procedures in an emergency room and you could do the same thing to this is that they offer people the G.I. cocktail. They don't know why and they've not figured out. Therefore, they suggest taken this G.I. cocktail immediately to determine whether it will ease the pain or not. The most common is an amalgamation of a liquid antacids, such as donnatal, often viscous lidocaine. It is an anesthetic used to aid in calming the burning and most often, if it will make people feel better immediately we believe that it is a heartburn, acid or reflux issue.

There's no 100 100% guarantee that you won't suffer from a heart condition since you can experience both. You could have a massive spaghetti meal, then experience heartburnand then suffer an attack on your heart and have a heart attack, therefore it's not a sure thing however, it can help reassure both the patient and the doctor, and means that we don't have to wait so long to see if symptoms get better. However, at home, you can experiment with homemade remedies such as liquid antacidslike Mylanta or chewable antacids and sometimes drinking plenty of water to ease things.

Some people utilize milk. Others may use a bit of alcohol and vinegar. You can also take non-prescription antacids, such as H2 blockers or Pepcid and many others often, they can assist you in determining whether you feel better immediately the reason is acid reflux. If you've had the same symptoms repeatedly and over and each time it is effective to use this type of medication, then it typically reduces your fear but many occasions, it could be more painful, or a new one, and it could be difficult to diagnose for a doctor or patient.

CHAPTER 2: WHAT CAUSES ACID REFLUX OR GERD?
Reason One - Stomach Contents

The traditional belief of acid also known as food particles are released in the stomach, occasionally even in the throat, and creates irritation and burning and that the lower esophageal and sphincter is the source of the issue. Another thing that could be causing problems is the excess stomach contents it could be due to the presence of too much food in the stomach. It is common for people to have an enormous meal, such as the spaghetti dinner or even a large Thanksgiving dinner, and consume plenty of food and then all the food is going down the stomach, and it sometimes is unable to find a place to go.

Therefore, you might not have enough space to put food into especially when it's a fat-rich, greasy food. The food may be less digestible and thus making it harder to take food items out of your stomach. There could be some inflammation, which can cause narrowing in the esophagus. Definitely should you put on your fancy dress that are tight slim clothes, and then to put lots of food in your stomach. It's likely to be squeezed into the stomach pushing the food up. If your food isn't being digested quickly enough, then wearing clothing which can fit your belly is essential.

Here's the image that we began with: the food is passing through the esophagus and it is now in the sphincter. It is affected, and acid is returning. The weak sphincter, therefore, is crucial and it connects both the stomach as well as the esophagus, and in the event that it isn't closed, the food will come back up and there are many reasons that people suffer from weak sphincter. A major and frequent causes is due to the age.

It is a pity to announce this in front of you. But it's that by the age of 50 60% of us are suffering due to a weak sphincter or suffer from hiatal hernias, or have some symptoms of reflux. Some people might not be suffering from symptoms. Some may even have erosion but not be aware of that they have it. Some may suffer from bleeding or even scar tissue. some may even develop cancer. There are patients who suffer from esophageal cancer which is a result simply by that constant acid that has been irritating the esophagus for many years.

Second Reason - Weak Sphincter

The hiatal hernia problem is an additional reason. It is the place where a tiny portion of the upper region of the stomach lies above the diaphragm's level which means that the fluids in the stomach sit higher than this and it is then reacted up. You can observe this in the image here. Another reason aside from the age factor and hiatal hernia, is being overweight. The greater the weight we carry in terms of stomach weight, the greater likely we're likely to put an increase in pressure on the stomach, that pushes things upwards which can cause weakness.

Image - Acid Reflux through the Relaxed Lower Esophageal sphincter

Here's a quick image of the sphincter that is relaxed and the acid flowing from the stomach into the esophagus. Then, hiatal hernia , as illustrated.

Acid Reflux resulting from Hiatal Hernia

Hiatal hernia isn't very often seen in children, however, we see it. It is definitely more prevalent as we age and become being overweight. Smoking is a risk cause. Sometimes , it is seen as a trend through families.

As you can see, a portion of the stomach's upper portion is situated above the diaphragm making it possible for acid to reflux easily. If you take a look at the image on the lower portion on the webpage, you will notice that there is a small balloon of stomach contents that is above the diaphragm's level. On the top image, the stomach is completely under the diaphragm. That's what they're trying to find when they use the upper G.I.

or scan to find out where the stomach is located when it's ballooned over the diaphragm.

Hiatal Hernia

This is the image from behind a bit and you can see a portion of the stomach above the the diaphragm. It's easy for the acid to rise higher than the sphincter, and eventually into the esophagus.

The traditional GERD Treatments, risks and Advantages

Acid Reflux Therapy

Let's discuss some of the most common treatments for GERD. They could include antacids, Maalox, Riopan, and Tum's. These may in certain patients cause constipation, diarrhea and muscle pains. Gaviscon is a well-known one that has magnesium and aluminum which is a form of a liquid that sits in the upper portion of the stomach. This means that whatever is coming into the stomach is not as acidic or neutralized, leading to less bleeding and burning, although it's sold over-the-counter, it should not be used during the pregnancy of a kidney or liver disease, or for the old who suffer from Alzheimer's.

It should also not be used if you suffer from or are taking Nizoral to treat a fungus, Tetracycline, or operating equipment that is heavy due to the possibility of nausea and dizziness and this could cause problems.

H2 (Histamine) Blockers

The H2 blockers now are something like Zantac as well as Tagamet. They are histamine receptor blockers and that's what H2 stands for. And initially , when they first came out they required prescriptions to obtain these. They do relieve heartburn, they also help reduce the acidity in the stomach. Now you can buy all one of them: Zantac, Pepcid, and other over-the-counter.

The issue can be the fact that Tagamet or Ranitidine is known to cause headaches dizziness, depression confusion, agitation along with central nervous system poisoning. So these drugs are not completely safe. In fact, Zantac or Ranitidine that is known as a generic term, may sometimes cause liver diseases, can cause harm or destruction to bone marrow. It can create anemia, cause white and red cells to break down and lead to breast enlargement.

There are women who want to have larger breasts however I'm not sure whether men have the same desire. Zantac can cause men to become impotent as well as muscle aches unclear vision and arrhythmia. Also, while these H2 blockers can be sold over-the-counter, it's not a guarantee that you won't experience issues.

PPIs as well as Magnesium Level Warn

These inhibitors of the proton pump are some of the most recent additions to the market and are very powerful and effective in blocking acid. That's the best part about. The most popular ones can be obtained easily - a lot of people use Prilosec which is also known as Omeprazole. This was the first , that was made available over the counter, but initially when it was released, there were a myriad of warnings about it being able to cause vision loss, and it may cause stomach cancer, and it's likely to be extremely risky but only take it for a period of two weeks.

However, now it is available over-the-counter and quite quickly. The most well-known is called the Purple pill that's known as Nexium extremely strong and extremely potent. However, it's costly, at least you need a prescription. I checked the cost on Rite Aid and if you decide to pay out of pocket it will cost you $293 for a thirty-day prescription. It's not cheap and the latest FDA warning, I believe it occurred two years ago recommends that you test your magnesium levels before and during treatment. Even when you are taking Prilosec or one of the other drugs, this testing is recommended since magnesium levels decrease and you're not getting magnesium, as well.

It's not just about causing muscle cramps and spasms as well as palpitations. If you're on heart medication, such as digoxin, and the magnesium levels are low, it could cause dangerous arrhythmias. Also, proton pump inhibitors are available over the counter and are readily available. Yes, you can use these drugs, but that doesn't mean they're not completely safe. They must be monitored.

Proton Pump Inhibitors

The proton pump inhibitors that are similar to Nexium and the purple pill and Prilosec are utilized to treat typical acid reflux GERD and in particular, in the case of the Barrett's Esophagus. Here's a photo of Barrett's esophagus. It is a serious inflammation and could be a prelude to cancer of the esophagus.

There are gastrinomas. These are tumors of the pancreas or duodenum that secrete gastrin which stimulates acid production. It can also occur in a different condition, Zollinger - Ellison Syndrome that can result in gastrin-secreting tumors in the pancreas. This, too, leading to a lot of ulcers and acid.

The most common adverse effects of proton pump inhibitors and I've met many people who can't take these side effects. include nausea, headache as well as abdominal pain, diarrhea and fatigue. They also experience dizziness and fatigue. In 2010 the FDA advised, and is in the document, not more than three weeks of treatment in a year. 14 days or 2 weeks for each of the PPI medications. Yet, the majority of people who take these drugs are taking them for several years in the same time.

PPIs and Images of Ulcerated Esophagus

Here's a quick image from inside, when you place an instrument in the mouth, and you're looking into the esophagus and you can see the muscles that are open in the lower esophageal sphincter which should be shut and you can see the red streaks, which indicate an ulcer caused by the acid that is leaking up into the esophagus due to that sphincter's not able to hold.

Here's a more appealing image of an stomach on the left. It's a pretty pink color and the sphincter appears to be shut, which is keeping acid from forming. On the other hand it is known as Barrett's esophagus. The sphincter is opened, and it's all bloody and inflamed. It's rawand generally receive regular scans every six months or year, to look for signs of cancer.

Barrett's Esophagus

Here's a second excellent image of Barrett's. Note the irritation and redness. Also, note the brutality of that acid that is leaking out, and this poses a risk. Therefore, we must reduce the risk as much as we can.

Acid Reflux Non Drug Therapy

Therefore, there are alternatives to drugs that you could explore in the event that they can help you, they're definitely worthwhile. They're a simple and safe method to do this, and to begin by avoiding big meals, and eat smaller portions each meal, and beware of eating food with a lot of grease and fat in it. This is because it's more difficult for this food to get through the stomach, which is why it is likely to be reabsorbed. Don't lie down within two hours after having an eating habit and do not wait until 10 pm to have your dinner and then lay down in the bed.

For some, when they lie on their backs and their sphincter does not shut off, their stomachs are in the air and their heads are down here and they're in certain to experience reflux. This means that for certain people even though there's been six hours between they last meal, they're still not safe to lay down. The beds we sleep in should not be flat, at least until we reach 50 years of age. Therefore, you can raise the bed's head with pillows. You could also make use of a wedge, and occasionally this works; you can also place bricks on the bed's head.

My favorite thing I say to people is to pull old blankets, pillows or towels from your closets, then lift your mattress. Then, place them between the springs and the mattress. So the entire top of your bed can be gently lifted up. No matter what the pillows are set or how you lay down your head, it is always higher than your stomach.

The second common thing to do is to stay away from smoking. Smoking cigarettes can cause irritation to stomach soft tissue which is a risk factor for cancer. The nicotine weakens the sphincter. It hinders it from closing and makes you more likely to have reflux. In addition, tight clothing or belts could increase the stomach contents and should be avoid.

Another reason to be cautious is if you are eating a large dinner and you're bent a lot or cleaning up and bending while playing tennis or golf or putting the balls down or taking them up, or engaging in any activity that puts pressure on your stomach, that is pushing that acid into your esophagus. Therefore, make sure to allow a bit of time between meals to begin.

Food-wise there are some foods that could be risky for some people, and this varies on the individual, are caffeine, chocolate and citrus, as well as onions and tomatoes. All of these can be problematic for certain people. Losing weight is an easy factor that can help many other aspects.

GERD Aggravator Chart

Again, this is an additional little summary and it lists triggers for heartburn such as alcohol, food soda, carbonated beverages pop, peppermint tomatoes, spicy food, and medications caffeine in coffee tobacco smoke, and other non-steroidal antiinflammatory's, and that's medications like aspirin Motrin, Aleve, Ibuprofen, Naprosyn and all the calcium channel blockers that are blood pressure medications in a plethora of ways - which means that a variety of substances you could be using that may be aggravating GERD as well as acid reflux.

Fundoplication Surgery to treat Acid Reflux

In the near future, I hope many of you will never need to undergo the procedure, however I was thinking that you may be interested in finding out the facts regarding the procedure of fundoplication. Fundoplication surgery is a solution to treat severe cases of GERD that are not controlled by medication or when patients do not respond to acid reflux medications.

It is the time when the surgeon removes an upper stomach loop to wrap it around the lower portion of the esophagus. They then sew it in place to create a kind of an extra muscle in order to stop the acid from that is coming back up.

This surgery helps strengthen the valve, which is the muscle between the esophagus as well as the stomach, and helps to prevent acid from returning to the esophagus. This aids in healing the esophagus, and in the event of a hiatal hernia is also repaired during this time. The positive side is that surgery can heal the inflamed esophagus for 9 out of 10 patients and eliminates reflux symptoms in 8 out of 10.

Here's a photo of a sketch that shows the place where they loop the muscle then tie it up and seal the loop...

...and I've also got a picture below of what it could appear like if you were actually there performing surgery with the upper portion of the stomach wrapped around the lower portion of the esophagus to provide an extra method of control.

The After the effects of surgery

The issue is, even though the surgeon could be a master at his job, after seven years of surgery, 4 out of 10 patients experience frequent symptoms of esophagitis or require medications or undergo another surgery. Seven years later surgery, two of the 10 experienced difficulty in swallowing and one patient was having difficulty swallowing.

Many feel the gas that they are unable to expel or swallow due to it being so small. Three out of 10 need to be taking medication, and typically, the reason people undergo surgery is because they can't endure medication. Additionally, vomiting could be difficult or even impossible to swallow and cause some irritation when you have the fundoplication procedure and it's not reversible or reversed, no matter what you do to alleviate the bloat or belch issues with swallowing and heartburn may be is, at this point you're stuck with these issues. It's therefore not something you want to take on - surgery is the last resort.

The holistic approach is the best option is the best option, and there's lots of literature by holistic physicians, claims that GERD is really a result of excess acid and is the reason for heartburn. The holistic doctors believe they could be able to pinpoint the causes however they are seeking answers to "Can acid deficiency cause similar symptoms?"

Their concern concerns "Are Acid blockers safe for long-term use as well as what will be the lasting impacts from the inhibitors of proton pumps and Prilosec?" We know from the research literature that B12 deficiency is extremely frequent, and the frequency of arrhythmias, muscular spasms and osteoporosis are extremely high when it is not in good condition.

What if these inhibitors of proton pumps create more acid when they are stopped? What are the other factors the reason why so many people suffer from heartburn, such as genetically modified food as well as electro-magnetic fields, food allergies as well as sugars and other food additives. What other triggers we should be aware of or avoid? And what are the natural remedies for heartburn?

For instance one of the natural GERD solutions I've had people attempt include eating organic

21

food, avoiding hormones and pesticides, avoiding excessive fructose corn syrup having a test for food allergies conducted, using EMF protections, which are for the electro-magnetic field and using specific minerals, herbs as well as essential oils, probiotics and stress relievers. A few of the stress-reducing substances could include biofeedback, the emotional freedom that is the way you can channel your feelings away, as well as testing for energy to let go of emotional blocks. There are many other alternatives to taking pills. I'm not saying that. I'm trying to convey.

Heartburn symptoms and acid production

Our bodies produce stomach acid as well as enzymes produced by the pancreas aid in digestion of food to break down the food that we are in a position to absorb all of the nutrients in the food, and we would like to maximize the benefits of the food we're eating, not just for the flavor. We also are aware that stomach acid is important in helping break down food items to absorb nutrients to ensure our long-term well-being.

If you decide to test someone, you can let them take small capsules. And there's an Heidelberg test that allows you to test how much acid is present present in our stomachs as we grow older. We can observe that the amount of acid isn't increasing with age. The issue is that from 60-65 There is a dramatic decrease in stomach acid which is detrimental to our health. We recognize that acid in the stomach is crucial for B12 levels, as well as for calcium absorption and magnesium absorption.

So, some of the symptoms experienced by those taking acid blockers for long-term, or people who aren't producing enough acid are that they may experience neuropathy, numbness, or tingling in their legs and arms, as well as confusion muscles, muscle weakness, spasms, osteoporosis and fractures, as well as macular damage which is very prevalent, and sometimes brain issues at the level of developing dementia. That's why acid in the stomach and at higher levels is crucial and could help in preventing these issues.

The low stomach acid is a sign of the aging process.

This chart outlines a small study studying the location of stomach acid is when it gets older. As it is evident that by the age of 60-69 50 percent of males and around five percent of females suffer from low stomach acid that, as we've mentioned earlier, is a problem, and is leading to weakness and neuropathy. dizziness as well as osteoporosis, confusion as well as mental confusion on and on on. Now, the question is "Why do we give the

23

people these antacids?" They need higher acid levels in their stomachs to be well, not lower.

Why low stomach acid can be an issue

We will discuss further about Hypochlorhydria that is a result of an acidity problem in the stomach, which is a serious issue which often is not diagnosed or treated. Most traditional doctors affirm that the stomach acid isn't all significant, and it doesn't play a significant part in breaking down food, and isn't significant in stimulating the production of pepsinogen in the pancreas. It is not a major issue and we do not really require it.

We also know that many health problems are caused by yeast and bacteria, particularly the harmful ones that are absorbed into our stomachs and system due to not having sufficient stomach acid. Also, we know that it's essential for all of the nutrition to break down and taken into our brains and bodies.

Although we're discussing excess stomach acid as being harmful and you're required to be taking acid blockers, we must admit it: stomach acid is essential for staying in good health for a long period of time. What's the difference in the views of traditional doctors and holistic doctors regarding the role of healthy stomach acid levels?

24

Hypochlorhydria as well as Heartburn

The best holistic doctors I've have read about are Jonathan Wright. He's a family physician along the West Coast, and he advocates for the actual test of stomach acid for patients who complain of heartburn. In addition, he claims that none of his patients who have visited him and have been treated with pron pump inhibitors or acid blockers has ever been examined. This isn't a standard thing that your doctor would like to examine. You're given an acid blocker, and you feel better, and the treatment ends there.

However, the fact that if you have lower acidity within the stomach the sphincter relaxes and this causes more acid, or whatever acid you've got, to rise back up, and then to back up into the stomach. The more acid you've in the stomach , the more it will help tighten that sphincter. This helps to absorb the food there, and keep it from returning up.

Relaxed Lower Esophageal Sphincter

The greater the damage to the sphincter gets and the more sensitive to food items and the condition gets worse. This is why we're concerned about that sphincter, and acid-reducing agents aren't helping and can make it worse.

They also relax that sphincter, and you'll experience an increase in symptoms. It just goes for a while, an endless cycle of symptoms and medication.

Reflux as well as Barrett's Esophagus

As we've said, acid blockers could reduce your symptoms as what's going on isn't as acidic, however there is more reflux, swelling, more inflammation in your esophagus greater stricture in the stomach, more cancer, more issues and Barrett's esophagus. Another thing which relaxes the sphincter food allergies. This is an individual thing for me.

Nearly every patient I've met suffering from heartburn for treatment, if I check them for IgG food antibodies, but not the IGE your allergist or dermatologist suffer from, like peanut allergies, they show food sensitivities. It's an IgG food allergy for gluten, wheat, eggs, dairy as well as corn, soy any of the usual ones. A minimum of 80% and sometimes nearly 100% of people suffer from a particular food sensitivity that if you eliminate the food you eat, your heartburn goes disappears.

I've seen this repeatedly and over over again. You don't require medication or to suffer from the side consequences.

The other option you can use if you're not taking melatonin is which can in tightening the lower esophageal sphincter. Certain people are able to sleep well as they age, while some don't, however, we know that Melatonin is depleted at the time you enter menopausal and, at age 50, it's very low. If you're not asleep in darkness at 10 pm at night, away from electrical devices, smart meters or mobile phone, the brain does not create melatonin. It does is not only tighten the lower esophageal sphincter which is beneficial, can also help your thyroid and your adrenal glands and helps you sleep better, and it lowers the risk of getting cancer in a dramatic way.

People who work at night and have very low levels of melatonin due to sleeping in darkness at night, have a greater risk of developing cancers of the colon, breast or prostate cancer. If you're not a high-risk patient for Melatonin, you'll have a higher chance of developing these cancers and if you're a cancer patient studies have proven that even in cases of severe metastatic breast cancers or lung cancers, as well as leukemia, if you provide the patient with the highest dose of melatonin, they will live two times longer than those who are not taking it. It's extremely potent. It is recommended to start doses at 3 mg, and for cancer, you could utilize 20-40 mg, which is the dosage. It's likely to be beneficial for anyone to take Melatonin, which is great for sleeping.

So , what's the problem with the acid reflux issue and Barrett's Esophagus - it's something that Gastroenterologists believe that once you've had the condition, it will be there for the rest of your life, and they'll continue to monitor you for a long time and wait until cancer symptoms develop and provide massive doses of acid blockers. Because of this, you'll have a relaxed sphincter and more food leaking out. This is a kind of catch 22.

A very important piece of advice is to have your body examined for food allergy like we discussed earlier when you're experiencing stomach acid or GERD symptoms. I haven't done an extensive study, however I've seen a number of patients who've visited an Gastroenterologist who told them they had Barrett's through biopsy, or could be unable to take anti-acid blockers because they made them sick , or they couldn't take them. They should avoid foods that appear in their tests for food allergies and their heartburn goes out and Barrett's esophagitis is gone and the next time it's back to normal! This is why I've witnessed this in many instances, which isn't heard of by gastroenterologists.

Security Risks from Acid Blockers

We'll go back to natural remedies and alternative therapies that are holistic. If you don't, you'll take these drugs and over-the-counter H2 blockers such as Pepcid, Tagamet, Zantac could be inappropriate for patients, particularly those who are 65 or older. All of these drugs are known to cause the decline of the brain in people who are elderly particularly those who have previously suffered from cognitive impairment. If you're starting to experience problems, these drugs could cause it to get worse. A study involving a huge sample of older African-Americans discovered that these blacks were 2.4 times more likelihood in developing cognitive loss which is the same as dementia and memory loss when H2 blockers were used constantly. That's a significant increase, 2 1/2 times the normal risk, and one of the things blockers reduce is the B12 levels in your blood which is the main cause of dementia.

It's true that many of us suffer from low B12 because of age, and the stomach acid doesn't have enough acid to take it in, even with the medications And then you add the drug and they really lower the B12 levels. Also, if you test your B12 levels and they say it's fine over 200, but 10% of people could suffer from neuropathy, neurological issues or depression lower than 400, then that's not a good sign, and in Japan they recommend that it be at or above 500. If you have B12 levels and you are a patient, inform your doctor that need to determine if it is not over 500. If it's not, you should take sublingual B12. Most people do not recognize that they have B12 levels that are low, and it's often the case.

ADVANCED SAFETY RISKS OF PROTON PHUMP INHIBITORS (PPIS)

We'll now discuss the dangers and security associated with proton pump inhibitors. which are the next category that is similar to Prilosec, Prevacid, Protonix, Aciphex, and Nexium the huge purple pill. They are extremely effective in stopping stomach acid and the problem we've talked about is that with low stomach acidlevels, it's not absorbing all of those nutrients, such as B12 as well as calcium and magnesium.

Another major worry is the chance of developing pneumonia. You don't consider the use of an acid blocker the cause of pneumonia however what they discovered is that if you're taking strong acid blockers, and the lower esophagus' sphincter is not in a relaxed state, that acid could be creating holes in the esophagus and leading to bleeding and ulcers, but also Barrett's and stricture, but in conjunction with that, while you're asleep, and you do not even be aware that this acid is redirected to the lungs and causes pneumonia.

This category of drugs, which they're referred to as PPI's or proton pump inhibitors comprise around 14 billion in sales for major Pharma pharmaceutical companies. It's also the top product in the sales for medications in the United States and some may require them, but some of us would consider other alternatives. The reason for this is that patients try to cut off all of these medicines and then suddenly the acid is not controlled. It is all of a sudden a massive increase in acidity in your stomach that says I'm back to work. And it's massive, and the sphincter is still in place and people suffer from horrible acid reflux and heartburn and say "Oh my god, I really require these medicines I must get back on these medications."

It's almost like an addiction. You begin to take these for a time and then it gets worse until you decide to take them. It's similar to being addicted to smoking cigarettes or cocaine or any other. This is why these companies have you hooked up to their profit-making machine in the form of selling their drugs.

Some of the more well-known negative effects or side effects of proton pump inhibitors are abdominal discomfort and diarrhea, fatigue and nausea as well as muscle spasm and pain as well as arrhythmia. Most of the time, people take these drugs and wouldn't ever think that a medication that blocks their acid will be the cause of these symptoms. There is no connection. You won't know until you stop taking them , what they could be doing, and what signs they might cause. Therefore, you must at least recognize that this could be the cause , and it could not be just you.

A recent study revealed that those taking PPI medications had a greater chance of contracting Clostridium difficile an extremely harmful bacteria that can be found in the intestine which can cause severe mucus, blood, diarrhea or pain, hospitalization, IV's that are intravenous, and this is a risk. In relation to the pneumonia, a research by Wake Forest University showed that cardiothoracic patients, also known as those with a heart or lung condition, who are prescribed anti-inflammatory drugs like Protonix, and the majority of the time , they take them at the ICU since they're concerned about stomach bleeding and stress ulcers. These patients were three times more at risk of developing chance of contracting pneumonia than patients who were not prescribed these medications.

The doctors think that they're doing a good job in trying to prevent the possibility of an ulcer or irritation, but they're also causing pneumonia. Moreover, giving these PPI medications resulted in an increase of 30% of death, as well as long and costly hospitalizations. Therefore, the final result is should not be the route you're looking for since there is a chance that you'll end in the hospital with pneumonia and then end up dying. It's true that you don't think that the use of an acid blocker was likely to be the reason of your pneumonia. However, the research showed that it could make an impact.

PPI Meds along with Osteoporosis

Another thing I'm worried about is osteoporosis. I'm aware of that the Canadian Medical Journal, not sure of the amount the AMA would be publishing it. They studied how PPI's were used in 65,000 patients This was a massive study that included people who were older than 50. The study found that over 15,000 people were who had osteoporosis-related fractures. This means that these patients were suffering from bone weakness Then they examined how many were taking these pron pump inhibitors over at least five years.

What they discovered is an increase of 62% in the risk of hip fractures caused by osteoporosis. Hip fractures can be painful and serious and can even be fatal. Most people spend the rest of their life in a nursing home in the event that they don't suffer from blood clots or pneumonia instead.

The hip fracture is a common occurrence is a possibility for some individuals. very well, but it's not something anyone would want to anticipate or even think about. If you are using the PPI's for more than seven years, it increases the likelihood of being injured in this way. Additionally it doubled the chance of all osteoporosis-related fractures and not just hips however, your wrist, the ankle, and spine, and else.

In other words, if you take these PPI's for an extended period of time and your body isn't capable of absorbing calcium, regardless of what calcium tablets you are taking or the amount of dairy you consume and drink, you're not going to be getting the magnesium, calcium, and B12 that your bones require and are likely to be weak.

Naturally, big Pharma says "We have a remedy for this, and we could offer you a second drug, such as Fosamax or something else." Therefore, take your Nexium first , and once you're eligible to be eligible for Fosamax and there's a chance that you'll get bone weakness , and all sorts of problems. This puts you in line to get more drugs, which is definitely not where I'd like to be. I'll point out that there are better alternatives that can help your bones. Boresha has a wonderful product to build bones, known as ARG Matrix and it is a product Boresha also a coffee maker, manufactures.

GMO Foods and Heartburn

Another thing to be cautious about are genetically modified food items. There's plenty of research and information going into this area, but we do know that when you consume GMO foods , they cause inflammation to the stomach. This could cause kidney failure and may cause tumors. The way they've approached this is to take animals like cows and pigs and fed them only pure genetically modified food. If you offer the food to them and then give them a choice to eat it, they will not take it. GM0 food. However, they eventually get hungry and will eat it even if they aren't given a option.

The pigs who did have an increased risk of 267% of stomach inflammation. Additionally, male pigs, for whatever reason, perhaps due to their diet, had a 400% increase in risk. It's interesting, but I'm not sure whether this is related to autism, but children with autism suffer from extreme stomach inflammation. Their stomachs and bowels are damaged, and we know that the majority autism sufferers are boys. There are some girls however, boys are more prone to it. Is this a correlation? perhaps?

The majority of corn that you consume within your diet in USA can be genetically modified. This is the corn-on-the cob your can of corn as well as your popcorn, corn oil as well as the sugar-free corn syrup which originates from corn and your corn chips. your corn cereals corn flour used in the majority of organic corn, you'll be able to find it however, most likely 95% of it is genetically modified, and they're not going to ever tell you that it's genetically altered and they'll fight it for years and don't need to disclose it to you. They don't inform you that it is not the case.

In addition, most soy consumed in the US is genetically modified. This is the case found in soy milk. I would strongly advise against using soy cheese, soy-based meats, is also used as a filler in variety of processed foods, in dressings and other products. Food industry uses it, along with the oil and protein in a variety of products that you aren't aware of and is harmful to your thyroid as well as inflaming your stomach.

The effects on the effects of Corn or Soy on pigs Stomachs

So I'm not sure what you see in the image, but this is a stomach of a pig, broken open and laid flat. The top portion is kind of light pink and flat There are no genetically modified foods that were consumed by the animal. The lower part is extremely inflamed, extremely rough, and extremely inflamed. the animal received genetically modified food.

Therefore, if the stomach is raw, you'll have more yeast, you're likely to have foods allergies. You're likely be diagnosed with cancer, you could experience all kinds of issues, and of course acid reflux. I'm not sure, perhaps it's a good idea to inquire with the pigs about whether they suffer from acid reflux, but I'm pretty certain they do.

Heartburn and food additives

Another thing to be aware of is the food additives. One of the experts I've often read includes the Dr. Russell Blaylock, who is a neurosurgeon, which means this guy is an absolute genius and is one of the leading experts on MSG as well as food additives. with his own newsletter and he has a warning for our government and these corporations do not care when you purchase more and require more, they'll throw it in simply because it's delicious. They also use aspartame and MSG to cause inflammation within your stomach, and in your digestive tract, and he's worried about your brain.

As neurosurgeons, he sees patients who have symptoms of brain inflammation, Parkinson's disease seizures, dementia or even passing out. the food additives cause ongoing inflammation, and cause damage to the brain, causing Alzheimer's disease, Parkinson's disease various things. Most of the time there is no indication on the label that it's MSG however, they list it in a different way and you must decide what you think it is as you please, and the wording could be something else, such as the autolyzed yeast (autolyzed), malt extract maltodextrin, hydrolyzed proteins, sodium caseinate or mono potassium glutamate, or textured proteins. If it doesn't say MSG and you don't have any idea of what is included as you're sure that most of us would like to work towards at avoiding Alzheimer's and Parkinson's disease the best we can.

Electro-Magnetic Fields as well as Intestinal Inflammation

A different issue to be concerned about today and more about electromagnetic fields. One among the people I spoke to, and also went through her book, was Elizabeth Plourde, PhD. Her website is www.emffreedom.com and also a book titled EMF freedom. She also talks often about how being in the vicinity of electromagnetic fields affects our health.

Wi-Fi is available, we've all had cell phones, and we have smart meters that are installed in our homes that they didn't bother us to discuss that are continuously transmitting radiation to us. It's everywhere you go. should you carry a smartphone in your head or even within your pants or on your stomach, wireless signal is causing microscopic inflammation in your stomach, your stomach, and your brain and you could experience headaches, suffer from dizziness, and you could develop food allergies, and you could develop brain cancer.

It is true that in the first 10 years being on the phone there is an increased risk of 25% of developing cancer in the brain. She found this out after they installed smart meters inside her neighbors' homes. Upon discovering this, she began to experience rashes and diarrhea and stomach pains and all the food she ate was absorbed by her. until she was able to shut off the smart meters from her and around her home , and repair her stomach and stomach, she was heading towards death. This book is fantastic. Also, EMF is yet another thing we've to be watching for.

Natural GERD Treatments and Holistic Doctors

Organic Honey Fresh Basil, Holy Basil Tea, and Indian Gooseberry

A few of the natural GERD solutions I'm going to discuss are organic and holistic foods and herbal treatments. One of them is organic honey that has not been refined that is inexpensive easy, accessible, and simple to sample, and can help reduce burning. The honey improves the pH and a amount at night can help reduce the intensity of burning.

Fresh basil is an Ayurvedic cure for acid reflux. Some have chewed on fresh basil leaves. However, you can purchase holy basil tea from the store selling health foods and Tulsi Tea, which is excellent for calming the body and Indian gooseberry, an herb that aids in protecting digestion by reducing stomach acid.

Licorice Root, Bromelain and Slippery Elm

Another one is licorice root. This helps to soothe as it forms the protective layer of mucus inside the esophagus. It is also available in tea form. can drink it in a tea form, simply monitor your blood pressure as it could rise occasionally. Also, Deglycyrrhized Licorice, which you can buy as a lozenge can be soothing and relaxing. Bromelain is an enzyme found in pineapple. Taking the enzyme or having a bite of pineapple before eating is a method to aid digestion of food you consume. It assists in moving food faster, so it's not sitting there for long.

The slippery elm plant is another one that coats stomachs like gooseberries that you can purchase and test. If you visit an health food shop,, you might come across these products or any combination that can be extremely beneficial Try one at a time to see how it affects your digestive system and the symptoms of acid reflux. Even if there are no symptoms, you should be aware of this fact - items that help your digestion can help you remain healthier and more youthful!

Cayenne Pepper, Apple Cider Vinegar and Baking Soda

Apple Cider Vinegar and Cayenne Pepper. Now, it's not easy to understand, but Cayenne pepper is used by some. It's a very hot pepper that you can put into water and it looks like it may burn, but there are people who have used it to ease inflammation and ulcers. It's the same is true for the apple Cider Vinegar as well as the organic vinegar. You add a small amount to water, and you believe it will be burning, but it can help to digest food and help move it through.

Additionally, you will are getting more nutrients from the food you consume. Apple cider vinegar might be the most simple, effective solution! Apply a few ounces prior to or after eating and especially if you are suffering from symptoms of heartburn. Watch disappear! Plus, for people who are elderly, it's giving acidity to the digestive system, which will help you absorb more nutrients into your body that you require including magnesium, calcium, and B12. This can help you prevent issues with your bones and also mental decline.

In the event of a need for short relief, you could bake soda in the yellow box but not the powder however, a point to mention here is that baking soda is an antiacid and, if you suffer from an acidic stomach as we age Perhaps it's best to incorporate an acidic ingredient to aid digestion, such as that of Apple Cider Vinegar so that we can get more nutrients from the food we consume. But baking soda is a great option to ease stomach pain.

Eat Slowly and Eat Smaller Meals

The most important thing you can do is chew their food in a slow manner. If you're eating your food, and you consume it slowly and chew it it will be digested some of it through the mouth's enzymes. When it's gone it's going to be much easier to pass through your stomach and start digestion faster.

Also, avoid big foods that are greasy and fat-laden; simply slow down to slow down and eat smaller meals slow down eating and you'll not be as likely develop acid reflux.

Digestive Enzymes

Another thing to take into consideration particularly if you're on the move for a long time, is digestive enzymes. It functions in a similar manner as Apple Cider Vinegar. Digestive enzymes are amazing and I have seen lots of people they aid. Our meals today are cooked or microwaved (I recommend you throw away your microwave, or only use it in the event of an emergency).

You can use some raw enzymes. As we age, we become less able to digest food. Therefore, if you are taking digestive enzymes in a supplement they can help in numerous ways. There are lots of excellent digestive enzymes available in the market, and they are extremely beneficial for helping to improve your digestion. You can also take them in capsules.

You can also take a bite of raw fruits and veggies. I've heard people say that they'll eat some pineapple, a small papaya, or a little pieces of raw Apple chew the fruit and then eat it slowly prior to eating and then have the enzymes to digest the food and help move it through. This is a very simple and affordable method and it's not anything more natural than that!

Probiotics

The other thing to consider is that when you're not having regular stool movements, then everything will begin to build up and cause stomachs to empty faster. Probiotics can help with this. They are fantasticand I believe everybody should be taking them. We need to maintain the beneficial gut bacteria in the stomach.

If you're drinking tap water that contains chlorine, it's making them sick, as is everything within the gut. And even if you're eating fermented foods that have been infused with good bacteria it, you're not replenishing it, and probiotics are the solution.

They are available as 25 or 50 billions in a tiny capsule and I really like the Chewables since they begin right in your mouth and get the bacteria. Yogurt, Kiefer, sauerkraut all of them help maintain the healthy bacteria levels in the right place and I truly believe that health starts in the digestive tract. It is vital for mental health. your mood may be affected.

What's the matter, there are numerous studies suggesting that if you're stressed, depressed or depressed, it is possible to take probiotics and be an effective way of making a difference! In addition, I like the Chewables but any way you can incorporate them is great.

There is no GERD Supplement

In terms of other supplements items I have tried There is one that's known as "No Gerd." It's a simple formula, and it makes use of d-limonene the organic substance, as well as some citrus fruits. The secret lies inside the rind. Even citrus peels are rich in it.

They are also known as Terpenes and Terpenes can be described as any of a group of hydrocarbons that are unsaturated including carotenes. They are discovered in the oils that are essential to numerous plants. They can help reduce acidity and heartburn as well as the acidity. This is among the methods I've used to help transition people off of the drug.

I start them off with an increased dose, possibly once a day. no GERD, and then taper off the H2 blocker and the PPI to ensure that it prevents that abrupt acid reflux rebound and also take this medication as a substitute to ease off the medication and then move to more natural ways of treating it.

There is no GERD is available through an online firm known as "Let's talk health" located in California and I keep it in my office. It is accessible over-the-counter. It's easy, it's easy to take, there is there is no toxic side effect that I am aware of and neutralizes stomach acid. As I mentioned, it's reliable and safe, as well as is low in toxicity, and has no adverse consequences. Another option that you can explore from your own.

Here's more information on how to use the No GERD formula, which is a method to wean patients off H2 and PPI Blockers.

Gastro Mend

Gastro Mend Another one I've used is from "Designs for Health" that is excellent Vitamin company. This one is a blend of a variety of products that I've used to treat stomach acid, as well as heartburn. Actually, I've seen many people treated for H pylori , without the need for an antibiotic. H Pylori is a very difficult bacteria to eradicate inside the stomach.

However, I've observed many who claim that Gastro Mend helped to treat. It contains mastic within it, and this has been utilized for many thousands of years throughout Europe, the Middle East and Greece, it's a plant, which is a gum that aids. It also contains MSM as well, deglycerized licorice and zinc carnosine. This is soothing, coats and heals and inhibits the growth of H. Pylori bacteria. I've experienced great results from the use of this.

This is how Gastro Mend looks like from the Designs for Health Company.

DoTERRA Essential Oil

Another feature doTERRA is the Essential oils business, offers is a product that you can buy as an oil, or in a capsule making it easy to chew and is made up of many things, including pepper, ginger and fennel. Caraway, Anise, and Coriander and essential oils.

Each of them has been utilized individually to treat intestinal disorders however, when combined and in a small pill, it's easy to treat heartburn and swallow it and help to soothe and calm your stomach efficiently. There aren't any reports of adverse effects from the product.

Acid Reflux Summary and Final

You may be aware or perhaps had the experience of certain foods can cause the symptoms of indigestion. Perhaps you had a hefty chocolate torte prior to bed and woke up days later feeling a simmering sensation in your throat and chest or perhaps a spicy meal caused you to need anti-inflammatory tablets a couple of hours later. A lot of people have had these experiences and know that at times, certain foods can cause heartburn.

There is a significant connection between the food you consume with acid reflux GERD or laryngopharyngeal respiratory reflux (LPR). There are three major methods that food items can trigger GERD and its variations:

* It could reduce the strength of the lower esophageal Sphincter (LES).

* It may increase acidity in the stomach.

* It may increase abdominal tension (IAP).

Acidity and alkalinity

Every substance has this property called pH which is a measure of alkalinity or acidity (or the neutrality). If you can recall the basics of science in high school, you will realize that the higher the pH of an item is, the more alkaline it is. Lower the pH is, the more acidic. The pH value of seven signifies that the substance is neutral. That is, it is neither basic or acidic. You may also have realized that the addition of an alkaline substance to an acidic one neutralizes its acidity.

The same principle applies for food items. If you suffer from an illness related to acidity levels inside your stomach for instance acid reflux, and other variations eating acidic food items to the system will increase the acidity. The addition of alkaline food items will help neutralize the acid.

Many people try to neutralize the acidity in their stomachs with antiacids, which are potent alkaline substances that could reduce stomach acids. However it is the International Foundation for Functional Gastrointestinal Disorders (IFFGD) mentions that, despite being rapid-acting, they're also only temporary solutions and could cause certain issues of their own like the possibility of rebound acidity (an rise in acidity in the stomach as a result of the use of these substances) and other adverse side effects that are not desirable.

However, eating foods with alkaline components does not carry the similar risks. For a permanent cure of acid reflux with no negative side negative effects, the best option is to opt for alkaline meals and avoid acidic foods.

Food Allergies, Sensitivities and intolerances

After rethinking my eating habits I found the one of my main Acid reflux triggers is due to food intolerances. What I realized was that when I ate food items that I was not tolerant I was more likely to experience acid reflux than if did not. It's because food sensitivities and intolerances impact your body's ability of digesting the foods you consume. Ingestion of these foods can cause problems which can cause an increase in IAP because they could...

* prolong the emptying process from stomach contents.

* cause poor or incomplete digestion.

* can cause gas and bloating.

* can cause changes in the gut bacteria (the microbiome of the gut).).

* can cause a condition that has symptoms that are similar to those of acid reflux.

Individuals may be intolerant or sensitive to a variety of common food items or components.

Gluten

As per "BeyondCeliac.org," about 1 percent of the population suffers from celiac disease which is an autoimmune type of gluten intolerance where sufferers are unable to process even tiny quantities of gluten. However, this percentage could be much higher, as experts believe around

83 percent of Americans who suffer from celiac disease are not diagnosed or mistakenly diagnosed. The group also estimates that 18 million Americans do not suffer from celiac disease however, they do suffer from gluten intolerance, also known as the non-celiac gluten sensitivities. Studies have found a strong correlation between the consumption of gluten by those who are intolerant and acid reflux-related events. In those with an intolerance to gluten (or celiac disorder) or acid reflux eliminating gluten is vitally essential to treat both of these conditions.

Dairy Products

People who are allergic towards dairy items (commonly caused by intolerance to milk sugar lactose, or an allergic reaction to milk's main protein, casein), GERD is often an underlying condition as per "Healthline." It's not just due to the fact that dairy products trigger GERD in and of themselves but because intolerances can trigger gas that raises IAP. Avoid dairy products when you're intolerant to it, particularly in the case of trying to manage acid reflux.

FODMAPS

Certain people are sensitive to one particular type of carbohydrates that are poorly digested, referred to as "FODMAPs" (fermentable polysaccharides (oligosaccharides) disaccharides, monosaccharides as well as polyols). These carbohydrates are present in various foods, from milk and fruit to beans and grains. For those with FODMAP sensitive, which usually manifests itself as irritable-bowel syndrome (IBS) eating these carbs can trigger an array of digestive symptoms, such as gas constipation, bloating, slow stomach emptying, and constipation, all of which could increase IAP and lead to GERD. When you've found yourself diagnosed with IBS or any other bowel disorders, such as Crohn's Disease, inflammation Bowel Disease (IBD) as well as colitis, you could be susceptible to FODMAPs within your food. For more details on FODMAPs and the best ways to stay clear of them, go to "Monash University" to find out more about the low-FODMAP diet to treat IBS.

Other Foods

It is also important to remember the fact that allergies to food can cause symptoms that may appear to be acid reflux, but can actually be the result of a condition known as "eosinophilic stomachitis" (EE). As per the Mayo Clinic, EE occurs when white blood cells are accumulated in the esophagus before becoming symptoms. Although EE is caused by acid reflux, the condition may have additional causes as an ailment caused by eating foods that cause an allergic reaction. The resulting inflammation can trigger various symptoms like GERD (or overlaps with it) like difficulty swallowing and chest pain that doesn't respond to anti-acids, chronic heartburn, and regurgitation.

If you suffer from GERD symptoms that do not respond (or do not respond in the same way you would like) to GERD medication or an acid-reflux diet, it could be that you have EE related to food or other substance allergies. Food allergens that are commonly found in foods that could cause EE are the most commonly used allergens - wheat, fish the peanuts, tree nuts dairy, eggs, and more uncommon allergies to foods. If you suspect that food allergies could be the cause of your symptoms, consult your physician about having tests done.

Foods that are a burden on the Stomach

N

All foods do not can have the same effect on digestion. But, there are certain foods which have been linked to acid reflux more often. These are usually foods are difficult to digest or those that alter the quantity as well as the acidity in stomach acids while they are processed. Pay attention to the presence of these foods within your diet and work to eliminate them or eliminate them entirely as much as you can.

Fatty Foods

The foods mentioned above, especially those that are fried and fried, are the most common cause for acid reflux. They trigger your LES muscles to relax, which allows stomach acid to get into the stomach. Avoiding foods that are fatty by those suffering from acid reflux issues as this can not only improve your LES function, but it will can also help you develop healthier eating habits that help in weight loss and fitness loss.

While you'll want to stay clear of the majority of fats, your body will require some fats to function. Make sure to choose more healthy fats, such as those that are naturally found in cooking oils or fish, like avocado oil or olive oil, when needed. Make sure to use these fats in moderation for maximum results.

Spicy Foods

Foods that are spicy are a frequent reason for acid reflux. Foods that are extremely hot and spicy usually contain an ingredient called "capsaicin," a naturally found source of heat in jalapeno peppers hot sauce, jalapeno peppers and other spices.

Capsaicin reduces the process of digestion giving acid reflux more opportunity when your body processes the food. Also eating food that's too spicy may cause irritation to your throat, causing more discomfort and damage. Avoid eating chili peppers, onions and garlic. In addition, limit the intake of black pepper to a minimum in order to lessen the symptoms of acid reflux.

Foods with acidic ingredients

Consuming foods that are acidic could increase the acidity that stomach bile is able to produce. Acid from the stomach that travels across into the LES and into the esophagus will be more likely to trigger an increased risk of acid reflux. To ensure that your stomach acid stays in the proper range of acidity eliminate low-pH food items out of your daily diet. It includes fruits with citrus, such as grapefruits, limes, lemons as well as pineapples and oranges. It is also recommended to avoid tomatoes. Acidity isn't limited to fruit. Sugars and refined grains are also considered to be acidic like some meat and dairy products.

If you're not planning to become completely vegan or gluten-free, think about reducing portions of those items you consume and replacing them with alternative options such as whole grains and protein sources that are plant-based.

Mint and Chocolate

If you're a huge chocolate lover, this could be a bit rough. Chocolate is rich in fat, and also has tryptophan, a chemical that triggers your brain to release serotonin. Although this may enhance your mood to some extent, serotonin as well as fat can loosen the LES muscle , allowing acid reflux to develop. Mint is also a great way to relax the LES. Beware of pain and stay clear of these desserts after dinner.

Drinks

The best drink to drink is water. option for treating acid reflux, and drinking drinks in general however, there are some drinks you must stay clear of. Anything high in caffeine can trigger acid reflux since they increase gastric acid. Tea and coffee are both acidic, and they can cause symptoms of acid reflux to get worse, just like the acidic juices of fruit or that contain sugar added.

It is best to avoid soda due to the carbonation that can cause digestive problems to worsen, as well as the sugar. Alcohol consumption may also cause acid reflux. Pure water, coconut water low-acid juices and smoothies as well as plant-based milk (like the soy or almond milk) are all safe choices for drinks.

Foods that aid in digestion Digest Better

T

The digestive process begins the first time you eat something. The saliva that you breath breaks down food molecules into smaller ones such as proteins, sugars and fiber. They break them down further and eventually turn into the nutrients required to support your health. Once you swallow these nutrients through the esophagus they're mixed with stomach acid and enzymes that make them a more sluggish liquid referred to as "chyme." The liquid flows through the small intestine, which is where the majority of the nutrients are absorbed prior to getting stored into the large intestine to be used for elimination through the feces or wastewater.

Certain foods can be helpful to help digestion. Here is a brief list of foods that aid us digest better.

Oatmeal

It assists in regulating the digestive system. it can treat diarrhea by making a paste out of oatmeal powder and milk and putting it on your stomach.

Water

It's beneficial for general well-being and can assist in softening stool and preventing constipation. Drinking chilled water or drinking at room temperature can have the same effect as drinking warm water.

Tomatoes

The tomatoes contain two kinds of fibers that can help increase stool movements. They comprise insoluble fibre (cellulose) and insoluble fiber (pectin). Soluble fiber absorbs liquids when it travels along the intestinal tract. It helps in softening stool and relieves constipation.

Yogurt

It is a good source of bacteria that produce enzymes which help digest food. The study took place by the University of Wisconsin (Madison) where those who consumed the most amount of yogurt experienced a significant increase in the number and amount of the bowel movements.

Wheat Germ

Wheat germ supplements have higher quantities of B vitamins and vitamin E. Both are essential to promote the growth and development of healthy bacteria within the intestines of your body. This improves digestion and can help fight colon cancer through its rich content in antioxidants, fiber Vitamin E, antioxidants, and other essential nutrients to maintain good health.

Bananas

Bananas are an excellent sources of fiber and are crucial to ensure regular constipation. The high mineral and carbohydrate amount of bananas assists in the production of healthy bowel movements. Due to their abundance of vitamins A and C they are great for your nails, hands and hair.

Watermelon Seeds

The seeds of watermelon contain a lot of antioxidants, fiber, magnesium, manganese and iron. This makes it a great digestive cleanser that will help treat constipation since it's rich in fiber.

Papaya Seeds

Papaya seeds are rich in the enzyme papain that is proteolytic which assists in digestion as well as alleviating the symptoms of flatulence (gas). It is also rich in vitamin B6 and Niacin. It is also one of the richest sources of vitamin A.

Broccoli

Broccoli has a chemical called "sulforaphane," which is well-known for its effectiveness in the elimination of harmful bacteria. Broccoli can also aid digestion and could help relieve gas, bloating and constipation, since it is a source of fiber.

Chia Seeds

Chia seeds contain mucilage that absorbs water from the digestive tract and releases it to soften stools and to lubricate the digestive tract. It also aids in reducing cholesterol and also in helping to prevent colon cancer, which is a common occurrence within the colon.

Garlic

Researchers have discovered 7 cloves per every day can cure the majority of cases of the condition known as halitosis (bad breath) caused by a chemical known as "allicin."

Nightshade Vegetables

The eggplants, tomatoes, potatoes peppers, solanum, and potatoes. These foods are rich in alkaloids "solanine" and "psoralens," which are potentially cytotoxic and have cancer-causing properties. So, it's best to avoid them.

Gastritis (The Fire Inside)

O

The stomach is protected by the gastric mucosal protection. It is based by prostaglandins. Prostaglandins play an essential function in preventing your stomach's lining burning by the acid it produces. As time passes, gastritis can develop because these prostaglandins are slowly diminished through:

* Excessive alcohol intake

* Infections caused by bacteria (such such as H. Pylori as well as "helicobacter Pylori")

* Certain medicines or steroids

* Stressful situations and stress at work and stress from relationships

* Anger that is excessive and long-lasting

* A weak immune system or an autoimmunity

* Acid Reflux Disease

* Long-term hostile behavior

Gastritis, as it is known, is a typical form of stomach upset, which causes irritation or erosion of the stomach's wall. In certain cases of gastritis, the lining the stomach can become inflamed or infected. In other instances the stomach's lining can become swollen or red In severe cases the inflammation could cause bleeding in the stomach and stomach lining.

Understanding the Different Types of Gastritis

The form of gastritis can be dependent on the severity of the condition and the underlying cause of inflammation. Thus, gastritis could be chronic or acute dependent on a variety of factors and the extent that the inflammation.

The acute gastritis inflammation is a serious disease that is usually due to food poisoning or eating food that has gone bad or just eating too much. In this instance the lining of your stomach can also become severely affected by the ingestion of harmful substances like poison acid, lye or poison. In cases of acute gastritis, two main complications could occur. These are commonly referred to as the gastric blockage and the pernicious anemia. Gastric obstruction, which is also known as "gastric outlet obstruction" is an inflammation of the deep tissues that can extend into the muscle in the stomach's lining and causes more inflammation of the stomach's outlet. The obstruction stops food from exiting the stomach and could result in vomiting , and the losses of electrolytes potassium, fluids and acids. However, pernicious anemia can occur when there is something that triggers burning of gastric parietal cells. These are the small cells that line the stomach.

The most common signs of acute gastritis comprise:

• Loss of appetite

* Feeling of fullness and pressure in the stomach pit (which doesn't get relieved by vomiting)

* Nausea

* Vomiting

* Headache

* Heartburn

* Fever

* Fatigue

A general feeling of illness

To combat acute gastritis, prompt medical attention is required and this calls for quick action by a doctor to eliminate the substance that is irritating. After the elimination of the substance, treatment might consist of neutralization of the substance that is irritating to prevent your stomach's wall perforating and causing acute peritonitis. In certain situations of severe gastritis surgery may be required. In general treatment for acute gastritis typically achieved within a few days after the removal from the irritating chemical.

Inflammation of the gastric tract is typically caused by the formation of an ulcer within the stomach. As previously mentioned there are numerous ailments that can cause repeated stomach irritations. The treatment time can be an extended period of time. In this case you may experience the sensation of feeling full after eating small portions of food. Contrary to acute gastritis that can be sudden the chronic form of gastritis develops at a much slower rate. The treatment for chronic gastritis is primarily by counteracting the large amounts of acid present within the stomach. By neutralizing the acidity levels of your stomach, you can aid in preventing further stomach liner erosion.

Extreme instances of Gastritis

There may be instances when symptoms of gastritis can be considered to be an emergency which demands immediate medical treatment.

Here are some severe gastritis signs that are believed to be urgent medical needs:

* Insueding swelling in the abdomen

* Stomach pain is getting more intense or shifting to the lower left abdomen (the appendix region)

• Frequent nausea (not not being able slow off liquids or food)

* Frequent diarrhea

Feelings of dizziness

* Stool with red blood

* Flickering

* Breathing difficulty

The pain can spread into the back, chest or neck or shoulders

• Vomiting blood (red or black)

* Condition keeping deteriorating

A

Acid reflux occurs when stomach acid builds up in the esophagus which is the food pipe. Acid damages the tissue of these organs and can cause irritation to your throat which can cause heartburns and unpleasant burps.

One of the main acid reflux triggers is food consumption. Acidic foods such as tomatoes and citrus fruits can cause this condition because they cause laxity in the muscles, which allows to digest and absorption into bloodstream, as per an investigation by Cornell University's On-Line Journal for Biosciences.

Certain foods aid in reducing the pain you could feel due to acid reflux. These are the following:

Beans

Beans are a great option for people suffering from acid reflux because they help ensure proper mixing of acids and bile acids in the body, which helps prevent stomach inflammation. It is crucial to keep in mind the fact that they are high in carbs or calories therefore, if you decide to turn to them as a food option make sure you have low-calorie food options as well.

Whole Grains

The dietary fiber that is found in whole grain and grains can be beneficial in stopping acid reflux as it helps keep food moving through the digestive system , without creating discomfort in the digestive tract. Make sure you're eating enough fiber-rich food frequently so that your body can absorb the nutrients.

Red Meats

Red meat is a rich source of protein, which can help increase an increase in the amount of hydrochloric acid within your stomach. This is how it helps to improve digestive system functioning. But, certain red meats are loaded with fat as well as cholesterol, which should be paid attention to, because they can cause harm to the esophagus due to rising acidity levels.

Fish

Fish contains omega-3 fatty acids. These help to prevent the stomach from being damaged. In certain instances the acids may cause excessive acidity in the stomach and the esophagus. It's important to ensure to include enough healthy fats into your diet, as they are vital to ensure the proper functioning of your brain and body.

Spinach

The fiber present in spinach may assist in reducing acidity levels in your stomach by helping to ensure that food items move through your system without a hitch and also provides nutrients necessary to ensure the normal functioning of your digestion.

Dark Chocolate

Dark chocolate is high in magnesium. This can assist you in addressing and preventing stomach acid reflux by helping regulate the muscles that propel meals through your stomach. This can help in reducing the severity of heartburn by reducing the amount of stomach acid.

Ginger

Ginger is abundant in anti-inflammatory properties, which trigger an increase in bile acid levels which are enzymes that naturally occur by the pancreas and the liver which help regulate and balance the quantity of gastric acid that is produced in the body.

Protein

Protein is essential as it aids in stop acid reflux through its ability to improve digestibility and the absorption of nutrients. It's also vital to release and produce of hydrochloric acids in your stomach.

Yogurt

Yogurt is beneficial for acid reflux as it helps in digestion so that foods can be reduced into small pieces and substances such as Bile will be easier to distributed across the entire body. Yogurt could also have probiotics to help fight stomach-related infections which can result from excess acid produced by the stomach.

Tips to follow at the table

For many for many, the phrase "acid reflux" signifies nothing. However, for those suffering from this ailment that is debilitating condition that causes eating to become an unavoidable social problem. Acid reflux is caused by stomach acid flowing up to the stomach. It can happen by poor posture or eating habits that creates excessive pressure on the stomach, and also when you lay down fast after eating, resulting the food being pulled by gravity upwards towards the throat and causes the stomach to produce more acid. Therefore, what do you do to stop this? Here are some important strategies to be aware of when you sit down at the table:

Keep Your Spine Straight Throughout Your Lunch (No Slouching)

It is crucial to be seated straight throughout your meal, and not slouch around the dining table. When you slouch and slouch, you place an extra weight on your stomach which could lead to stomach acid or heartburn. Therefore, not lie down as soon as you finish eating and to maintain your head at a in line in relation to your entire body during the meal. This will stop stomach acid from accumulating in your stomach , and then entering your esophagus. This creates severe discomfort and pain.

Eat slowly

Although eating slowly can lessen the effect of eating too much it is crucial to not eat so fast that you don't fully take in or chew. You might think that you're eating slow however in reality that you could be eating so fast that you're not spending the time take a bite and take a swallow. This could cause indigestion and result in excess stomach acid build-up within your stomach. This creates discomfort and pain in the stomach.

Chew Well

According to a study those who don't chew effectively during meals have more frequent acid reflux. If you don't chew properly, food becomes stuck in your throat. This can cause extreme irritation and pain when stomach acid builds up.

Eat at least three hours before bedtime

Food eaten prior to bedtime or just before falling asleep has been found to affect your ability to sleep and lower the quality of your sleep. If you consume food too before the time you go to bed, your body is likely to focus more on in digestion rather than sleeping, which can lead to a poor quality sleep and sleepless nights. Therefore, ensure that you don't eat for at least three hours prior to going to go to bed. This will to ensure you get an excellent night's sleep and will feel rejuvenated early in the day.

Avoid Alcohol

Alcohol can cause acid reflux to become more severe, as evidenced by several studies. Furthermore, it is recognized to boost levels of stomach acid. It is therefore recommended to stay clear of drinking alcohol at the beginning of meals that are acidic. If you do decide to drink alcohol, it's best to restrict the amount you consume and be careful about how you consume it as there can be negative effects that could result from drinking excessively.

Beware of sharks and Tuna Fish when packing

Do not eat tuna fish for 2 hours prior to bedtime, as it could cause heartburn as tuna fish is a source of lots of mercury that can affect the way your body process food. This can result in more sodium in your stomach than you need. It's okay to consume tuna fish 2 hours prior to the time you go to bed. Therefore, you should avoid these meals entirely when you're about to sleep.

Beware of Dairy Products Before Bedtime

The lower levels of dairy products within the body can cause the symptoms of acid reflux as well as indigestion that can also increase the chances of developing the reflux condition, GERD, or heartburn. It is advised to avoid dairy products before you go to bed because they can cause stomach upset and trigger acid reflux. However, it is acceptable to consume the occasional consumption of dairy products like cottage cheese, yogurt or melon, during the day, if you would like to are not exposed to the bacteria that can cause illness.

Reflux and the Way to stop the Fire The rising

from the stomach

G

Astric acid reflux isn't an ongoing condition It is common for people to experience it after eating a certain food. It's normal in a variety of situations, and it is able to be reduced or eliminated by using certain natural or medical solutions. If it's not properly treated or if a person has a digestive issues it can become ongoing and get more severe. The chronic illness of acid reflux is known as gastroesophageal conditions. It typically occurs in people who constantly feel acid or food leaking through the tube of the canal that connects the throat and stomach. It's also known by the name of "heartburn" and causes discomfort, as well as other possible risk to the health of a person. In this situation the patient is able to feel or experience the unabsorbed stomach contents or food in the food tube as well as in the throat. It could cause damage to the inner tube's lining as well as the stomach's walls too.

Acid reflux can quickly affect people with any other health problems. It is frequent in people who have both Type 1 as well as type 2 diabetes. Patients with asthma can also be affected by acid reflux. A poor digestion, or any other stomach-related disorders can cause acid reflux. The treatment for this issue is essential to take place in time to avoid other health problems If it is not addressed it could lead to numerous serious complications.

According to research, it has been proven that acid reflux may be caused by poor eating habits and the consumption of too many fried foods or carbonated drink. This may weaken the ability for the stomach to absorb food quickly and also make it hypersensitive to it. Other health issues may be the cause of the gastric acid reflux. In the beginning of the condition, which is caused by the low concentration of diet as well as lifestyle adjustments, the issue is easy to treat and managed before it turns into an actual problem.

Treatment for Acid Reflux

In the wake of unhealthy lifestyles and unhealthy habits which can cause a variety of health issues which include acid reflux as one of the most common. Our lives are often busy, and it's difficult to locate "time" to take a meal in time "right timing." This can lead to poor eating habits and can lead to improper eating times. This can increase the weight of an individual and could cause weight gain. These actions directly affect the quality of your sleep and your mind. If you don't feel calm and is feeling agitated digestion is one of the more sensitive component of the entire body. The digestive system is the first to feel the effects of stress first. This can lead to poor digestion of food and can cause acid reflux.

According to medical doctors and health experts acid reflux is a medical issue that can be treated and, with the help of a few modifications to your lifestyle, it could be conquered easily. For the treatment of acid reflux, the primary factor to consider is diagnosing the condition. The first suggestion is that foods you aren't allowed to eat include the fried and fatty foods including canned and processed foods carbonated drinks, alcoholic drinks as well as citrus and pepper. These foods can trigger heartburn , and cause restlessness and may cause irritation or even damage.

In addition to the restriction on food and the food restrictions, it is important to cut down on the amount of the meals that is consumed by a person in the course of a day. A big meal will fill your stomach, causing an increase in the reactions or irritation. With smaller meals the stomach may have plenty of space which means this can reduce the amount of reflux. Additionally, it is essential to consume the final meal three hours prior to going to bed and therefore, avoid eating meals prior to bedtime.

To prevent the condition from becoming worse To prevent the condition from recurring, you should keep your head in a straight line to your body while you lie down. This assists in controlling the flow of acid or food to the stomach and reduces the heartburn that occurs at night. Don't use a large pillow as it exerts stress or pressure on your stomach, which can cause an unrestful state.

As you make lifestyle and dietary changes , continue to talk with your doctor and take medications as well. The medications can help reduce the impact of reflux or stop the acid reflux from having an adverse effect for your overall health.

Complications due to Acid Reflux

Acid reflux can be a digestive condition that can be managed by taking medication or changes in lifestyle. However, if it is not treated correctly and if the issue remains untreated for a prolonged period of time the condition can impact the stomach as well as other body organs as well. It's a backflow or reflux in stomach acid, or the flow of food toward the food canal that causes heartburn. Because of the movement of the fluid inside the throat, one might experience discomfort and dry cough, too. Someone suffering from gastric acid reflux typically feels chest pain that can be described as heart-related, however it's actually due to gas and the effects of reflux, which is caused by the stomach. The symptoms can get worse when not treated promptly. Acid reflux can cause damage to the lining of the esophagus and could cause bleeding too. This can cause ulcers in the stomach or be persistent over time. In the case of insufficient treatment for stomach acid reflux It is also observed that some suffer from the ongoing issue of narrowing their esophagus liner. In time, it may be the reason for cancer of the esophagus as well. This serious condition can not only cause health issues for the patient, but could also cause a reduction in activities or decreased productivity. In the worst case scenario it could even be life-threatening. The best way to prevent these issues is to focus on a minor issue and seek the appropriate treatment from your health professional promptly.

If you're in the beginning stage of acid reflux, it is essential to be aware of your lifestyle. By making small adjustments to your diet and lifestyle an individual will not be able to just get over the problem, but also receive the care they require on time. With the help of natural foods and home remedies, it's simple to treat and manage acid reflux. It is all you need to do is be aware of acidic or unhealthy foods that can increase the acidity of the stomach. Eat food that is low in salt and spices. This helps to reduce the irritation. Also, take small meals portions all day long. We also have recipes to assist you in making delicious meals that will provide relief from acid reflux too.

Common Symptoms

P

eople are prone to the classic signs of heartburn as soon as they eat. Foods that are large and greasy and spicy, as well as starchy can be more troublesome. The symptoms are more severe when you eat fast or lie down or exercise shortly after eating. When you have the silent reflux (LPR) the signs are either constant or intermittent. They can occur during meals or in between meals, throughout the day or at night.

They are the most frequently reported symptoms of reflux GERD and LPR.

* Heartburn

* Regurgitation

* Chest pain

* Breathlessness

* Hoarseness

* Trouble swallowing

* "Lump" sensation in the throat

* A choking sensation

* Chronic cough

* Clearing the chronic throat

* Postnasal drip

* Trouble breathing

* Airway obstruction intermittent

* Heezing

The index of symptom severity for reflux (RSI) above is a diagnostic tool created by Drs. Jamie Koufman and Jordan Stern which can assist you in determining whether you suffer from LPR. It's not meant to replace a full medical evaluation and diagnosis, however, it can help you identify the symptoms you're experiencing and how severe they're. Scores of 15 and more indicates that you have LPR. However, when you're not able to get a higher score and you suspect you might have it, it's recommended to speak in with an ENT specialist.

In the past month what was the most significant issue have you been affected? (0-5 score, where zero means no problem , and 5 indicates a serious issue)

Problems with your voice. 2 3 4 5.

Clearing your throat 0 2 3 4 5.

Postnasal drip 5 5

Trouble swallowing liquids, food or pills 0 2 3 4 5.

It is common to cough after eating or upon lying down. 1 2 3 5

Chesting episodes or breathing problems 5 5

A sour or irritating cough 1 2 3 5

A feeling of something sticking in your throat. 2 3 4 5.

The chest hurts, you have heartburn stomach acid appearing to be 5 5

Total

Tips for treating flare-ups in an emergency

If you're experiencing heartburn that is causing you to flare up You can try one of these treatments:

* Ginger: to improve digestion, prepare ginger-infused tea, by adding 1 tablespoon of fresh

grated ginger with 1 cup of warm water. Add 1/2 teaspoon of maple syrup, if you want.

* "Aloe vera" Plant: You might be familiar with Aloe vera beverages in the stores However, these drinks tend to include sugars and preservatives. Instead, put aloe leaves in your fridge or cultivate an aloe plant at home. Cut an aloe piece and then remove the hard , green skin leaving the transparent, gooey portion. Blend it into a drink.

* Bone broth: Sipping warm bone broth may help to soothe the throat's lining as well as the your esophagus.

* Get up: or If you're lying down lift your head up using pillows, so that your body is elevated above your body.

* Take a break If you're doing work or running other chores, relax for a few minutes to slow down. Relax for five minutes and breathe deeply.

* Walk It Off If you've had a bad day and have a hangover, take an easy walk. Avoid jumping and any other exercise which involves too much shaking.

When do I need to see an ER Doctor?

When you've already tried the eating plan and changed your diet up to 4 weeks, and you still experience symptoms, you might want to consult a gastroenterologist, as well as an ENT (otolaryngologists) physician. They'll be able to test for a variety of disorders, ranging from Barrett's Esophagus to cancerous ulcers and ulcers. If you're suffering from a serious problem the earlier you recognize it, the greater your chance of achieving an entire recovery.

If you are suffering from at most one of these symptoms it is recommended to make your appointment with a physician sooner rather than later.

* Heartburn severe that occurs more than two times per week, despite adhering to the recommendations in this guide and/or taking prescription medications to suppress acid for more than 2 weeks

* Extreme chest pain after eating, which appears to be an attack on your heart (this is usually a reason to make visit to your gastroenterologist, however of course, chest pain can be a sign of a heart attack when it's coupled with other symptoms of heart attacks like pain or tension in the neck or arms, lightheadedness, a erratic heartbeat or anxiety, immediately dial 911.)

* A severe cough that keeps you up in the late at night (especially when it's so intense that you fear you'll be suffocated or out of breath)

* A cough that lasts for longer than 3 months, regardless of normal chest Xrays and rule out any throat or chest infection

• Pain, or discomfort swallowing, a choking feeling or a continuous feeling of an unsettling swelling in your throat

* A ringing in the morning that becomes worse during the daytime, or a shaky voice

* Feeling of obstruction or narrowing in the esophagus.

* Vomiting or nausea (especially when vomiting blood, since it may be a sign of an esophageal ulcer)

* Stools with blood or black stool movements

In order to help your doctor determine an appropriate diagnosis, make a note the symptoms you experience, the time they occur, as well as the degree. Note down when, when is happening, and the amount you take in. Monitoring your stress levels and sleeping patterns will help you understand the way your environment influences your symptoms. The symptoms you experience will likely improve, however in the event that there isn't, your physician will want to know why.

The results of medical tests and doctor's appointments can be unpleasant or even stressful. However, eliminating more serious medical issues will ease anxiety and let you concentrate on making and eating nutritious meals. If tests reveal negative results it will be possible to begin treatment earlier and will have a better chance of success.

The Most Important Causes

There is no one specific reason for acid reflux, it could be a combination of or more causes. It is the job of a doctor to assist the patient in identifying the possible causes and formulate an appropriate treatment strategy. We will investigate a variety of possible causes before coming to any conclusion.

The most basic, well-known reason for acid reflux is due to the production of excessive acid in the stomach. When food is absorbed into the stomach it triggers an acid release to break down the food into smaller pieces. The amount of stomach acid released will depend on the amount of food consumed and the kind of food item needs being broken down. For instance, low-fiber food items and sugars that are simple (like refined flour and other products) are easily reduced to their smallest forms and don't require a lot of stomach acids to break down. Complex particles, such as animal proteins and high-fiber food may require greater amount of acid in order to break them into smaller pieces.

If this recognition system goes out of line it could cause stomach acid that isn't suitable with the type of food. If a large amount of acid dissolves food item, it's removed from the stomach to the small intestine. If the stomach continues producing acid in an empty stomach, it's likely to create problems. If there is too much acid produced, symptoms of reflux are more likely to develop.

Pharmaceutical companies thrive off this idea, since there are numerous prescriptions as well as non-prescription remedies that function to reduce stomach acid. The idea behind this suggests that if there was less stomach acid in general and less stomach acid, less entering the esophagus, thereby reducing the symptoms, and also causing lesser harm.

Functional Issues that can lead to GERD

There are also a variety of functional issues that affect the stomach and esophagus that could lead to acid reflux. When food is ingested into the mouth and then slides into the esophagus, before reaching the stomach the lower esophageal muscle (LES) is opened to allow the food bolus (chewed chunk of food) into the stomach. and then it closes swiftly behind the bolus, securing the esophagus from acid that attempts to get into. The LES is precisely adjusted to close at the precise moment that the bolus enters it. Should there be confusion with the signals or there is nerve damage, like or a swollen nerve, the LES might begin to expand at unintentional times and allow stomach acid to pass through the esophagus.

The lower esophageal muscle can also be damaged or bent that prevents it to fully close. It could be an issue of structural nature or stomach problems. When there is a rise in abdominal pressure, this presses upwards over the lower esophageal and sphincter and opens it up a bit. If the seal of the sphincter is damaged and any acid that splatters through it could cause burning or an unpleasant sensation, commonly referred to as heartburn. In excess food intake within the stomach can lead to pressure, mostly due to eating too quickly. It is also possible to have an issue with the stomach, causing it to drain slower which allows food to accumulate and cause pressure.

Hiatal hernias are another possible reason for frequent reflux. Hiatal hernias occur when there is a bigger than normal opening inside the diaphragm, where the esophagus extends to join the stomach. This space is large enough to allow the stomach to protrude out and put tension on your lower and sphincter. There is a good chance of acid in the esophagus.

Hiatal hernias can develop in the beginning or over time. It can vary in size, which can cause different signs. The majority of hernias are benign and are not noticed until the doctor suspects that it could be the reason behind the symptoms. Changes in diet can help with the majority cases, however surgery can be a solution to more severe cases.

Acid Reflux and Stress

Stress appears to be the most frequent cause of body-related ailments. It can trigger headaches that can turn into migraines, cause muscular aches, fatigue hypertension, as well as other issues, such as acid reflux as well as GERD. According to a study from 2011 published in "Healthline," there is an undisputed correlation between work-related stress and the development of GERD. Participants reported a higher incidence of GERD when they were under stress. The study was conducted in Norway which included more than 40,000 people. They also found that job satisfaction levels were low. an underlying theme.

Another study conducted in 1993 found that anxious people experienced a greater intensity of symptoms than those who were more relaxed. Incredibly, the study showed there was no connection between these higher anxiety and a noticeable rise of stomach acid. This suggests that stress has an influence on the receptors within tissues' cells, which increases their sensitivity to stimuli and creates the appearance of more symptoms. The researchers believe that stress causes sensory receptors within the brain, triggering more of an emotional reaction than could normally be caused by a tiny amount of acid within the esophagus. The findings show that symptoms can appear exaggerated in stress-related situations.

It is important to note that the subjects in this study had already experienced signs of acid reflux. the study was designed to find out the impact of stress and signs of GERD. The study doesn't suggest that stress is the cause of acid reflux, but that symptoms could be more severe when stress is present.

Additionally the studies are confined in the sense that they've examined the effect of stress-induced acid reflux, such as exposure to cold temperatures or loud and annoying noises in controlled settings. They didn't test the effects of chronic, continuous stress that is often due to strained living environments or financial issues, illness or chronic problems in the workplace. While there are some acute stressors but the majority of people are suffering from chronic, long-term stressors that are deep-seated in time.

Although no earlier studies showed an rise in stomach acid because of stress, an interesting study from 1990 showed an association between stress-related rises the amount of acid in your stomach. It discovered that people who have certain traits in their personality respond differently to stress and this reaction either increases or reduces your production of stomach acids. They discovered that people who tend to be laid-back and analytical are more likely to lower stomach acid levels when they are exposed to stressors that cause acute anxiety. However, those who are more emotional and faster to react, have higher acid in their stomachs when stressed is present. This suggests that there's something else that is causing acid reflux and stress however the reason for this is not yet clear.

For a different perspective that is involved, recognize that breathing patterns change in response to stress. While a relaxed and calm person can take long deep breaths, someone in stress may breathe shallowly and in short bursts. This response is long-standing in humans have existed since. When faced with stress that is acute that is known as"the "fight or flight" response early on, humans needed to boost the amount of oxygen that entered the body in order to prepare for a "fight or flee" scenario. When faced with the threat of death or danger it is common for the heart rate to increase and breathing speeds up in order to increase the oxygen supply to the muscles which include the heart. It is an uncontrollable bodily function, and you have no control over it, unless you know that it's taking place and conscious try to regulate your breathing.

The negative side effect of breathing shallowly is a weakening in the muscles around the lower esophageal muscle. Deep breathing permits these muscles to stretch out to their fullest as they contract. Breathing shallowly only uses an insignificant amount of muscle capacity to perform. It's similar to doing a bicep curl at the gym only flexing the muscle half way. The entire muscle is not being worked out, and as a result it will weaken as time passes.

This is a great theory to explain how stress causes acid reflux. When stress levels are high the chance of breathing in shallow breaths is increased. The muscles that surround the lower esophageal muscle shrink which leaves the lower esophageal muscle unsupported and open to letting in unwelcome stomach acid.

Bacteria and GERD

New research is starting to identify the microbiome, an assortment of numerous beneficial bacteria that reside within the gut, and to be the cause of pressure. It is understood that the various bacteria, known as"the "gastrointestinal systems home" generally provide various functions to our body for space. Bacteria help in the digestion and absorption of minerals and vitamins and aid in the regulation of the digestion process. Healthy, non-harmful strains bacteria that live in large colonies aid by keeping the smaller colonies of harmful bacteria under control. They are an extension of your immune system. This is the reason why yogurt is advised to assist in digestion problems. The microbes present in yogurt culture helps to increase the number of beneficial bacteria that live within the gut, thus aiding digestion and ensuring the population that are harmful to bugs.

Bacteria feed on a variety of elements however the most sought-after are sugars that are broken into carbohydrate-rich food items, like pasta, bread and fruits. Since the bacteria consume those nutrients, they generate gas as an end-product. The more sugars that are simple to digest the greater amount of gas the colony produces. The gasses have no place to go other than up, before being absorbed by the stomach and increasing pressure. The lower esophageal muscle is opened to ease pressure, it allows the gastric acid from the stomach enter which damages the lining of the esophageal.

Although beneficial bacteria aid in helping the body to break down food items, harmful strains such as Helicobacter Pylori (H. Pylori, for short) causes more stomach acid made and can cause the symptoms of acid reflux. Human bodies have a long record of being exposed to H. Pylori and can be cured of it. H. Pylori is sensitive to stomach acid and thrives in an alkaline or neutral environment. The body releases more of stomach acid due in the presence of bacteria. H. Pylori is a hard bug to eliminate therefore stomach acid levels are typically elevated for longer durations which causes frequent reflux symptoms. When cells of the stomach are subjected to higher levels of acid than they are used to over a prolonged period and peptic ulcers start to appear. If not treated the ulcers will begin to bleed, and then the blood is leaking out of the body. If the condition persists, nutritional deficiency and other major issues occur due to losing blood. In addition that this condition can be very painful. Stabbing, shooting pain is a frequent complaint. Along with stomach acid-reducing drugs patients are likely to require antibiotics to aid the body in fighting against H. Pylori infections.

Pregnancy

Acid reflux is a common occurrence by women in their first pregnancy because of the increase in pressure caused by the growing fetus addition to the increased hormonal levels. The highest level of acid reflux is during the third trimester and the signs of acid reflux begin to fade disappearing shortly after the birth.

Smoking

Alongside increasing the risk of developing cancer of the esophagus adverse consequences of smoking are believed to be the cause of acid reflux:

* Enhanced secretion of acid

* Reduction in muscle function LES

* Reduction in saliva production (saliva is effective in neutralizing acid)

* Mucus membranes damaged

* Impaired reflexes of the throat muscles

Diet

Sleeping on the couch immediately after having eaten or eating an extra meal could cause heartburn as well as many other signs associated with acid reflux i.e. difficulties with food swallowing dry cough, and so on.

The following foods that are commonplace are known to trigger acid reflux:

* Carbonated drinks

* Alcohol

* Foods that are spicy, e.g., chilies and curries

* Chocolate

* Tea (with tea leaves) or coffee (including both regular and decaffeinated)

* Citrus fruits, i.e., lemons, oranges, etc.

* Foods that are fried or rich in fat.

* Garlic and onion

* Foods that contain tomato, e.g., pizza or salsa, as well as spaghetti sauce

There are a variety of causes of acid reflux, including:

* Obesity and obesity

* Eat a healthy meal prior to bed

Consuming more food and following that, either bent to the side or lying down in the bed

• Consuming muscles relaxants different medication to lower BP (blood pressure) and even Ibuprofen and aspirin, for example.

Foods to be affixed as preferred

What to Eat

T

The following foods can aid in managing the symptoms of acid reflux. If you notice that you are experiencing acid reflux Try eating at least one of these food items to alleviate your symptoms. Don't be discouraged if you take a bite of something and you don't notice a significant difference. In the end, you'll discover the food that works the most effectively for you.

Vegetables

We all recognize that vegetables are healthy for us. To be honest adding more vegetables to your diet can boost the quantity of nutrients your body gets. They naturally are low in acidity and fats. A good choice is the leafy veggies, greens broccoli, cucumber and cauliflower.

Ginger

Do not think that you need to gobble down on a full thumb of ginger. Luckily, you don't require a large amount to reap the benefits. One method of incorporating ginger into it is adding some sliced or crushed pieces into your smoothies, food items or meals. It is also possible to prepare ginger tea. Ginger is a food that has natural anti-inflammatory properties and is excellent for a variety of digestive issues.

Oats

Anything that is high in fiber can benefit the digestive system and may aid in relieving acid reflux. Oats are simple to prepare and are loaded with fiber. It is easy to incorporate into your daily diet by eating it for breakfast along with fruits.

Non-Citruscitrus Fruit

Fruits are generally extremely beneficial for your health, so it will benefit your body when you increase the amount of fruit you consume. Citrus is rich in acid which is the reason why you should stay clear of these kinds of fruits. A few of the fruits you can add to your diet include bananas, melons, apples and the pears.

Lean Meat and Seafood

The word that is most crucial in this case is lean. These kinds of meats have low fat, and are high in protein. The most common examples include turkey, seafood and chicken. Grilling them or poaching and baking is the best option. Beware of burning them.

Egg Whites

The egg itself is full with protein and nutrients, however, the yolk is packed with fat. This can trigger acid reflux. Restricting yourself to only whites is an excellent method to get the protein and avoid the fat.

Healthy Fats

Healthy fats can help in the treatment of acid reflux. It's trans and saturated fats that can cause a serious issue. Although it's not recommended to consume large quantities of any kind of fat, healthful fats are full of nutrients and may help reduce acid reflux symptoms. The sources of healthy fats are avocados, nutsand flaxseed and olive oil.

What Drinks to Drink?

We've all heard that beverages high in caffeine, acidic beverages, and carbonated drinks aren't ideal for those suffering from acid reflux. But, we've not yet spoken about the kinds of drinks you need to consume. Don't forget this. It is important to avoid drinking too much liquids since this can trigger your acid reflux symptoms to worsen However, some drinks are extremely beneficial for you.

Herbal Teas

Herbal teas are fantastic to aid digestion and can be commonly used to treat digestive problems of all kinds. The licorice, chamomile, as well as ginger are most effective for acid reflux. They ease stomach pain and help soothe your stomach. Be sure to stay away from mint teas.

Smoothies

These are definitely a fantastic method to incorporate more nutrients to your diet. The great thing is you are able to include ingredients that can aid to ease your stomach. Apples, bananas ginger, citrus, and other non-citrus fruits are excellent choices. Smoothies are simple to digest and are easy to swallow and cool when they're consumed. Drinking a smoothie that contains all the ingredients you need can ease with acid reflux and symptoms.

Fruit Juices

We've talked about the need to avoid the consumption of citrus fruits However, citrus fruits aren't the only fruits that produce fantastic juices. There are many non-citrus fruit which can also be juiced. One of the best ways to obtain your juice is to use cold-pressed juices. They retain their nutrients and are not contaminated by unneeded flavors and ingredients. You can purchase them at the markets or buy an juicer and then juice your own fruits and vegetables. The best options include ginger, carrots aloe Vera, watermelon and cucumber.

Water

We must all incorporate enough water in our food intakes. The PH level of water can be neutral meaning that it could help increase the acidity of a food. Consuming too much water could result in adverse effects for acid reflux. Therefore, make sure you don't drink too much. If you drink it when you're thirsty, you'll be fine.

Food Swaps

Food swaps are among the most effective ways to transition into a new lifestyle or lifestyle. There are many foods we love and it is difficult to let go of certain foods. Food swapping lets you make use of something similar to substitute of the items or foods you love. Let's look at some of the food swaps that you can incorporate into your daily routine.

Coffee to Herbal Tea

There are plenty of coffee drinkers on the planet, however, the caffeine in coffee is harmful for those suffering with acid reflux. If you're still in the market for an enjoyable warm drink opt for the herbal varieties instead. They are more gentle to stomach and a lot of them actually aid digestion. You can add milk to make more creaminess if you aren't satisfied with the water and tea.

Once you're comfortable with tea, you'll never feel the need for coffee. It's an issue of going on until you don't want coffee. Keep in mind that caffeine is addicting, which is the reason that so many people have a hard time letting go of coffee. If you're one of those who drink coffee many often throughout the day, it is possible that you will need to remove yourself from it or experience some withdraw symptoms prior to you are able to eliminate it. Don't get discouraged when it's difficult in the beginning. It will pass and you won't be able to remember it.

Citrus Fruits for Berries and Melons

The reason why so many people love citrus fruits is that they're so delicious and sweet. There are many other fruits with the same qualities. They might not taste identical, but melons and berries are both juicy and tasty. Make sure to fill your fridge and baskets with them instead of the citrus fruits.

I'd go as going as to say that melons and berries are superior to citrus fruits when it comes to availability and variety. It is possible to cook with berries more easily and incorporate into dishes. Making them into garnishes or toppings is a good idea. Smoothies made from this fruit are delicious. The options are limitless.

Chocolate to Carob Powder or Alkalized Cocoa

I think that the thought of giving the chocolate we love can make many who suffer from acid reflux extremely sad. Everyone loves a chunk of chocolate. But the problem is that chocolate is also high in fat as well as acidic. It's an additional trigger. That is why it's best to not eat it when you are suffering from acid reflux. If you can get the block without creating heartburn, then absolutely try it. Be careful not to overdo it.

If you're in dire need of chocolate fix, consider carob powder or alkalized cocoa. Alkalized cocoa can also be referred to as Dutch-processed cocoa which is more acidic than alkaline. This makes it suitable for those suffering with acid reflux. Carob powder is not connected to cocoa and is derived directly from carob pods. It is very similar to cocoa and can incorporate it into recipes that call for cocoa.

But, it's not an excellent idea to pick up a teaspoonful of these powders and consume it in one go. They'll have a bitter flavor. They should be added into the food. Chocolate desserts and cakes are made with either of these two methods, and should satisfy your craving for chocolate.

Fried Food to be used for Baked Food

Fried foods are generally unhealthy for anyone, even if you don't have acid reflux. The high fat content contributes to weight gain, and can also trigger acid reflux. It is recommended to cut out all fried foods a miss and attempt to eliminate out fried foods from your diet in the maximum extent you can.

It is possible to bake almost everything you fry. Because it's the method of cooking that has changed in this case, you don't need to alter the foods you eat. There are a lot of recipes that can transform ordinary foods into nutritious baked and healthy alternatives.

High-Fat Dairy Products for Plant-Based Options

Dairy products can also be frequently a trigger for acid reflux. It's an extremely difficult thing for people to let go of since it's almost an everyday item in everyone's kitchen. There is good news that there are many vegan alternatives to dairy. They can be found in supermarkets, and a lot of them aren't very expensive .

Alternative milk options include almond milk, soymilk and Oat milk. Instead of regular yogurt, opt to coconut yogurt. It is possible to use all of them as alternatives to dairy products that are commonly used. This makes it simple to add to your favourite recipes. If you're searching for a cheese substitute it is possible to find vegan cheese. It's more expensive than normal cheese. If you're looking for some cheese in your meal you can choose this. It is also possible to include a little nutritional yeast to give a cheese-y flavor to your meals.

Tomato Pasta Sauce for Pesto

The tomato sauces that are served with pasta are a classic, however this isn't the only method to take advantage of pasta. Pesto is an excellent method of eating pasta and it's delicious. You can also drizzle olive oil on your pasta for a lighter recipe. Pasta is delicious with many things, so don't be trapped because you're giving that red sauce pass. You can also make the low acid tomato sauce recipes from this book if are in the market for tomato paste. It's a fantastic method to taste the red sauce, too. Be careful that you don't overdo the sauce because not all of acid is neutralized.

Garlic and Onions for Dried Versions

Though they're not consumed by themselves however, they can provide a variety of flavor to food. Most dishes call for either or both of them, and it is difficult to make a tasty dish without these two ingredients. Instead of using fresh onions and garlic Try using dried versions. These are much less likely to trigger acid reflux. The benefit is the fact that it doesn't need to chop garlic or breaking onions while you cook your meal.

There's a chance that dried varieties could still trigger you. If that's the case, consider using different spices and herbs for flavor. Dill, basil and parsley provide lots of flavor to many recipes. They don't taste as much as onion or garlic However, that doesn't mean you won't be in a position to create a delicious tasting dish with them.

Alcohol as a substitute for alcohol that isn't alcoholic.

Alcohol is an acid-reflux trigger therefore it is advised to stay clear of the drink completely. If you're mildly sensitive, you may be able to enjoy a few drinks. Be careful not to go overboard. It is essential to be aware of the limits of your body as it is your health that is your most significant aspect.

If you like drinking a glass of wine on occasion there are alcohol-free options that are suitable for you. It is still recommended to stay clear of carbonated drinks, which is why it's not an excellent idea to consume alcohol-free champagne or non-alcoholic beers. Instead, try non-alcoholic wines and mocktails (which are similar to regular drinks however without the alcohol). In all likelihood it's not necessary to have any alcohol to live your lives. It's not a necessity and you shouldn't think that you're missing out on something since you don't get to enjoy a drink.

WALLS

1. Cinnamon Apple "Fries"

Prepare Time 10 mins

Timing of Cooking: 12 Minutes

Servings: 4

Ingredients:

2 red apples cored, peeled, then cut in wedges

* 1 tbsp. melted coconut oil

* 1 tbsp. pure maple syrup

* 1 tsp. ground cinnamon

* A pinch of sea salt

Directions:

1. Pre-heat the oven to 375 degrees F.

2. Prepare a baking sheet by covering it by using parchment.

3. A large mixing bowl mix together the coconut oil, the apples and cinnamon, maple syrup and salt until they are evenly coated. Place the apples on a single sheet over the sheet you have prepared.

103

4. Bake for 12 minutes and until apples have been cooked.

Nutrition:

* Calories: 98

* Fats: 2g

"Saturated Fat 2 grams

* Cholesterol 8 mg

* Carbs 19 grams

* 3 g fiber. grams

* Protein: <1 g

* Sodium * : 60.1 mg

2. Bacon Wrapped Melon

Prepare Time 10 mins

The cooking time is 0 Minutes

Servings: 4

Ingredients:

* 1/2 cantaloupe with rind removed, seeded and rind removed and cut into 8 wedges

* 8 extremely small Canadian bacon slices

Directions:

1. Cover each melon wedge with one piece Canadian bacon and secure them using toothpicks.

Nutrition:

* Calories: 28

* Fats 1 grams

"Saturated Fats: Zero grams

* Cholesterol 7 mg

* Carbs: 2g

* Fiber 1 grams

* Protein: 3 g

* Sodium 302 mg

3. Honeyed Mini Corn Muffins

The preparation time is 5 Minutes

Cooking Time: 15 mins

Servings: 12

Ingredients:

1. 3/4 cup cornmeal

* 3/4 cup all-purpose flour

* 1 tbsp. baking powder

* 1 tsp. baking soda

* 1/4 tsp. sea salt

* 1/2 cup of unsweetened almond milk

* 1/4 cup honey

* 2 eggs, beaten

* 2 tbsp. canola oil

* 2 tbsp. nonfat plain Greek-style yogurt

Directions:

1. The oven should be preheated to 425°F.

2. Line a mini muffin Tin with mini cupcake liner.

3. A medium-sized bowl is used to mix together the flour, cornmeal baking soda, baking powder and salt together.

4. In a separate bowl, mix the almond milk eggs, honey, eggs oil, and yogurt.

5. Mix the wet and dry ingredients together, and mix until it is just together. The muffin cups should be filled with 1/2 to 3/4 full.

6. Bake for around 15 minutes up to the point that a toothpick stuck into the middle is clear.

Nutrition:

* Calories: 217

* Fats: 11g

106

"Saturated Fat": 7. grams

* Cholesterol 27 mg

* Carbs: 28 grams

* Fiber 2 grams

* Protein: 4 g

* Sodium: at 167 mg

4. Buttermilk Biscuits

Prepare Time 15 mins

Cooking Time: 15 mins

Servings: 8

Ingredients:

* 3/4 cup all-purpose flour

Whole wheat flour, 3/4 cup

* 1 tsp. baking soda

* 1/2 tsp. sea salt

* 2 tbsp. cold butter that is unsalted and not seasoned Cut into pieces small enough to be able to cut

* 1/2 cup nonfat plain Greek-style yogurt

* 1/4 cup buttermilk with low-fat

* 2 tbsp. honey

Directions:

1.   Preheat the oven to 425°F.

2.   Line a baking sheet with parchment paper.

3.   In a medium bowl, whisk together the flours, baking soda, and salt.

4.   Using two knives or a pastry blender, cut in the butter until the mixture resembles coarse oatmeal.

5.   Stir in the yogurt, buttermilk, and honey.

6.   Drop the dough in 8 equal portions onto the prepared sheet. Shape them lightly into rounds.

7.   Bake for 14 to 15 minutes, or until golden brown.

Nutrition:

•   Calories: 138

•   Fats: 3 g

•   Saturated Fat: 2 g

•   Cholesterol: 8 mg

•   Carbs: 24 g

•   Fiber: <1 g

- Protein: 4 g

- Sodium: 317 mg

5.   Baked Tortilla Chips with Black Bean Dip

Preparation Time: 10 minutes

Cooking Time: 15 minutes

Servings: 4

Ingredients:

- 4 corn tortillas, cut into 8 wedges each

- 1 tsp. sea salt, divided

- 1 (14-oz.) can black beans, drained and rinsed

- 1 tsp. ground cumin

- ½ tsp. ground coriander

- 2 tbsp. fresh cilantro, chopped

Directions:

1.   Preheat the oven to 350°F.

2.   Line a baking sheet with parchment paper.

3.   Spread the tortilla wedges in a single layer on the prepared sheet. Sprinkle with ¼ teaspoon of salt.

4.   Bake for about 15 minutes.

5.   Meanwhile, in a medium saucepan over medium-high heat, warm the black beans, cumin, coriander, and the remaining ¾ teaspoon of salt for 5 minutes, stirring occasionally.

6.   Transfer the mixture to a blender or food processor and process until smooth. Stir in the cilantro and serve with the warm tortilla wedges.

Nutrition:

- Calories: 393

- Fats: 2 g

- Saturated Fat: 0 g

- Cholesterol: 0 mg

- Carbs: 73 g

- Fiber: 16 g

- Protein: 23 g

- Sodium: 485 mg

6.   Jicama with Low-Fat Ranch Dip

Preparation Time: 10 minutes

Cooking Time: 0 minutes

Servings: 8

Ingredients:

- 1 cup fat-free cottage cheese
- 1 cup fat-free sour cream
- 2 tbsp. fresh dill, chopped
- 1 tbsp. fresh thyme, chopped
- 1 tsp. fresh chives, chopped
- 1 tsp. lemon zest, grated
- ½ tsp. sea salt
- 1 jicama, peeled and sliced

Directions:

1. In a medium bowl, stir together the cottage cheese, sour cream, dill, thyme, chives, lemon zest, and salt. Serve with the sliced jicama for dipping.

Nutrition:

- Calories: 90
- Fats: <1 g
- Saturated Fat: 0 g
- Cholesterol: 5 mg
- Carbs: 14 g
- Fiber: 4 g
- Protein: 6 g

- Sodium: 262 mg

7.　　　Baked Green Bean "Fries" with French Fry Sauce

Preparation Time: 10 minutes

Cooking Time: 15 minutes

Servings: 4

Ingredients:

- Nonstick cooking spray
- ¾ cup bread crumbs
- 1 tsp. dried thyme
- ½ tsp. dried rosemary
- ½ tsp. sea salt
- ¼ tsp. ground cumin
- 2 eggs, beaten
- 1 tsp. Dijon mustard
- 1 lb. fresh green beans, trimmed and halved
- 1 cup French fry sauce

Directions:

1.　Preheat the oven to 425°F.

2.	Spray a baking sheet with nonstick cooking spray.

3.	In a large bowl, mix the bread crumbs, thyme, rosemary, salt, and cumin.

4.	In another large bowl, whisk the eggs and mustard together.

5.	Add the green beans to the egg mixture and stir to coat.

6.	Toss the coated beans with the bread crumbs to coat. Place them in a single layer on the prepared sheet.

7.	Bake for about 12 minutes, or until golden brown. Flip and bake for 3 minutes more. Serve with the dipping sauce.

Nutrition:

•	Calories: 100

•	Fats: 2 g

•	Saturated Fat: <1 g

•	Cholesterol: 43 mg

•	Carbs: 13 g

•	Fiber: 3 g

•	Protein: 8 g

•	Sodium: 607 mg

8.   Baked Potato Chips

Preparation Time: 5 minutes

Cooking Time: 25 minutes

Servings: 4

Ingredients:

•   Nonstick cooking spray

•   1 medium russet potato, cut into ¼-inch-thick slices

•   2 tbsp. extra-virgin olive oil

•   ½ tsp. sea salt

Directions:

1.   Preheat the oven to 400°F.

2.   Spray a baking sheet with nonstick cooking spray.

3.   In a large bowl, mix the potato slices, oil, and salt to coat. Spread the chips in a single layer on the prepared sheet.

4.   Bake for about 25 minutes, or until crisp and brown.

Nutrition:

•   Calories: 131

- Fats: 7 g

- Saturated Fat: 1 g

- Cholesterol: 0 mg

- Carbs: 16 g

- Fiber: 2 g

- Protein: 2 g

- Sodium: 237 mg

9.   Sweet Potato Oven "Fries"

Preparation Time: 5 minutes

Cooking Time: 25 minutes

Servings: 4

Ingredients:

- Nonstick cooking spray

- 1 medium sweet potato, cut into ¼-inch-thick strips

- 2 tbsp. extra-virgin olive oil

- ½ tsp. sea salt

Directions:

1.   Preheat the oven to 450°F.

2.   Spray a baking sheet with nonstick cooking spray.

3.   In a large bowl, mix the sweet potato strips, oil, and salt to coat. Spread the fries in a single layer on the prepared sheet.

4.   Bake for about 25 minutes, or until crisp and brown.

Nutrition:

- Calories: 101

- Fats: 7 g

- Saturated Fat: 1 g

- Cholesterol: 0 mg

- Carbs: 9 g

- Fiber: 2 g

- Protein: <1 g

- Sodium: 244 mg

10.   Maple-Thyme Roasted Carrots

Preparation Time: 10 minutes

Cooking Time: 20 minutes

Servings: 4

Ingredients:

- Nonstick cooking spray

- 4 carrots, peeled and cut lengthwise into quarters

- 2 tbsp. extra-virgin olive oil

- 1 tsp. orange zest, grated

- ½ tsp. sea salt

- ½ tsp. dried thyme

- 2 tbsp. pure maple syrup

Directions:

1. Preheat the oven to 400°F.

2. Spray a baking sheet with nonstick cooking spray.

3. In a large bowl, mix the carrots, oil, orange zest, salt, and thyme to coat. Spread the carrots in a single layer on the prepared sheet.

4. Bake for about 20 minutes, or until the carrots are brown and roasted.

5. Toss with the maple syrup before serving.

Nutrition:

- Calories: 118

- Fats: 7 g

- Saturated Fat: 1 g

- Cholesterol: 0 mg

- Carbs: 15 g

- Fiber: 2 g

- Protein: <1 g

- Sodium: 277 mg

11.   Roasted Parmesan Potatoes

Preparation Time: 10 minutes

Cooking Time: 20 minutes

Servings: 4

Ingredients:

- Nonstick cooking spray

- 2 cups Yukon Gold potatoes, diced ½-inch pieces

- 2 tbsp. extra-virgin olive oil

- ½ tsp. sea salt

- 1 tbsp. fresh rosemary, chopped

- 2 tbsp. Parmesan cheese, grated

Directions:

1.   Preheat the oven to 450°F.

2.   Spray a baking sheet with nonstick cooking spray.

3.   In a large bowl, mix the potatoes, oil, salt, and rosemary to coat. Place the potatoes in a single layer on the prepared sheet.

4.   Bake for about 20 minutes, or until crisp and brown.

5.   Toss with the Parmesan cheese before serving.

Nutrition:

- Calories: 113

- Fats: 7 g

- Saturated Fat: 1 g

- Cholesterol: 0 mg

- Carbs: 12 g

- Fiber: 1 g

- Protein: 1 g

- Sodium: 271 mg

12.   Mac 'n' Cheese

Preparation Time: 15 minutes

Cooking Time: 5 minutes

Servings: 4

Ingredients:

- 3 cups (1 recipe) low-fat white sauce

- 2 oz. fat-free sharp Cheddar cheese, grated

- 6 oz. whole-wheat elbow macaroni, cooked according to package directions and drained

- 1 tbsp. melted unsalted butter

- ¼ cup bread crumbs

Directions:

1. Preheat the broiler to high.

2. In a medium saucepan over medium heat, cook the white sauce and Cheddar cheese for 2 to 3 minutes, whisking constantly until the cheese melts.

3. Add the hot macaroni and toss to coat. Divide evenly among four (6-oz.) ramekins, or spread into a baking dish.

4. In a small bowl, mix the butter and bread crumbs. Sprinkle over the mac 'n' cheese.

5. Broil for 1 to 2 minutes, or until the bread crumbs are golden brown.

Nutrition:

- Calories: 258

- Fats: 5 g

- Saturated Fat: 2 g

- Cholesterol: 14 mg

- Carbs: 41 g

- Fiber: 4 g

- Protein: 12 g

- Sodium: 343 mg

13.   Quick Rice Pilaf

Preparation Time: 10 minutes

Cooking Time: 10 minutes

Servings: 4

Ingredients:

- 2 tbsp. extra-virgin olive oil

- 1 carrot, peeled and cut into ¼-inch dice

- ½ apple, peeled and cut into ¼-inch dice

- ¼ cup slivered almonds

- 1 tsp. dried thyme

- ½ tsp. sea salt

- 1 cup cooked brown rice

- ¼ cup vegetable broth

Directions:

1.　　In a large sauté pan or skillet over medium-high heat, heat the oil until it shimmers.

2.　　Add the carrot, apple, almonds, thyme, and salt. Cook for about 5 minutes, stirring occasionally until the apples and carrots are soft.

3.　　Stir in the rice and broth. Cook for 5 minutes more, stirring occasionally.

Nutrition:

- Calories: 290
- Fats: 11 g
- Saturated Fat: 2 g
- Cholesterol: 0 mg
- Carbs: 43 g
- Fiber: 4 g
- Protein: 5 g
- Sodium: 295 mg

14.　　Mushroom and Pea Couscous

Preparation Time: 10 minutes

Cooking Time: 5 minutes

Servings: 4

Ingredients:

- 1 tbsp. extra-virgin olive oil

- 1 cup sliced mushrooms

- 1 cup peas, fresh or frozen

- 1½ cups vegetable broth

- ½ tsp. dried thyme

- ¼ tsp. sea salt

- 1 cup couscous

Directions:

1. In a medium pot over medium-high heat, heat the oil until it shimmers.

2. Add the mushrooms and cook for 5 minutes, stirring occasionally.

3. Add the peas, broth, thyme, and salt. Bring to a boil.

4. Remove from the heat and stir in the couscous. Cover and let sit for 10 minutes. Fluff with a fork.

Nutrition:

- Calories: 240

- Fats: 5 g

- Saturated Fat: <1 g

- Cholesterol: 0 mg

- Carbs: 40 g

- Fiber: 4 g

- Protein: 10 g

- Sodium: 410 mg

15.   Simple Sautéed Greens

Preparation Time: 5 minutes

Cooking Time: 10 minutes

Servings: 4

Ingredients:

- 2 tbsp. extra-virgin olive oil

- 4 cups chopped kale, or other green of choice

- 2 tbsp. vegetable broth

- 1 lemon, zested

- ½ tsp. sea salt

- A pinch ground nutmeg

Directions:

1.   In a 10- or 12-inch sauté pan or skillet over medium-high heat, heat the oil until it shimmers.

2.   Add the kale, broth, and lemon zest. Cook for 5 to 10 minutes, stirring constantly until the kale is very soft.

3.   Season with the salt and nutmeg. Serve immediately.

Nutrition:

- Calories: 95

- Fats: 7 g

- Saturated Fat: 1 g

- Cholesterol: 0 mg

- Carbs: 7 g

- Fiber: 1 g

- Protein: 2 g

- Sodium: 287 mg

16.   Mixed Veggie Stir-Fry

Preparation Time: 5 minutes

Cooking Time: 6 minutes

Servings: 4

Ingredients:

- 2 tbsp. extra-virgin olive oil

- 1 cup mushrooms, sliced

- 1 cup peas, fresh or frozen

- 1 carrot, peeled and diced

- 1 cup broccoli florets

- ½ tsp. ground ginger

- 2 tbsp. gluten-free soy sauce

Directions:

1. In a 10- or 12-inch sauté pan or skillet over medium-high heat, heat the oil until it shimmers.

2. Add the mushrooms, peas, carrot, broccoli, and ginger. Cook for about 5 minutes, stirring frequently until the veggies are soft.

3. Stir in the soy sauce. Simmer for 1 minute more.

Nutrition:

- Calories: 110

- Fats: 7 g

- Saturated Fat: 1 g

- Cholesterol: 0 mg

- Carbs: 10 g

- Fiber: 3 g

- Protein: 3 g

- Sodium: 499 mg

17.   Guacamole

Preparation Time: 10 minutes

Cooking Time: 0 minutes

Servings: 6

Ingredients:

- 2 avocados, peeled, pitted, and chopped
- ¼ cup fresh cilantro, chopped
- 2 tbsp. fat-free plain Greek yogurt
- ½ tsp. ground cumin
- ½ tsp. lime zest, grated
- ½ tsp. sea salt, or to taste

Directions:

1.   Combine all the ingredients in a medium bowl. Mash and mix with a fork until the avocados are mashed and the ingredients are well blended.

Nutrition:

- Calories: 101
- Fats: 9 g
- Sodium: 202 mg
- Carbs: 5 g

- Fiber: 4 g

- Protein: 2 g

18.   Avocado Deviled Eggs

Preparation Time: 10 minutes

Cooking Time: 0 minutes

Servings: 4

Ingredients:

- 4 large hardboiled eggs, peeled and sliced in half lengthwise

- 2 tbsp. fat-free plain Greek yogurt

- ½ avocado, peeled, pitted, and mashed

- 1 tsp. orange zest

- ¼ cup fresh tarragon, chopped

- ½ tsp. sea salt

Directions:

1.   Use a spoon to scoop the egg yolks from the whites. Put the egg yolks in a small bowl and put the whites cut-side up on a platter.

2.   Add the yogurt, avocado, orange zest, tarragon, and salt to the egg yolks. Mash with a fork and mix.

3.   Spoon or pipe the mixture into the egg halves.

Nutrition:

- •   Calories: 123

- •   Fats: 9 g

- •   Sodium: 358 mg

- •   Carbs: 4 g

- •   Fiber: 2 g

- •   Protein: 8 g

19.   Roasted Fennel

Preparation Time: 10 minutes

Cooking Time: 40 minutes

Servings: 4

Ingredients:

- •   2 fennel bulbs, cored and cut into pieces

- •   2 tbsp. olive oil

- •   ½ tsp. sea salt

- •   ½ tsp. grated lemon zest

Directions:

1.   Preheat the oven to 400°F.

2.   In a large bowl, toss the fennel with the olive oil and salt. Spread in an even layer on a rimmed baking sheet.

3.   Bake until the fennel begins to brown, about 40 minutes, flipping after about 20 minutes.

4.   Toss with the lemon zest before serving.

Nutrition:

- Calories: 96

- Fats: 7 g

- Sodium: 352 mg

- Carbs: 9 g

- Fiber: 4 g

- Protein: 2 g

20.   Honey-Roasted Carrots

Preparation Time: 4 minutes

Cooking Time: 40 minutes

Servings: 40

Ingredients:

- 2 cups baby carrots, halved lengthwise

- 2 tbsp. olive oil

- ¼ cup honey
- ½ tsp. sea salt

Directions:

1.   Preheat the oven to 400°F.

2.   In a large bowl, toss the carrots with the olive oil, honey, and salt. Place in a single layer on a baking sheet.

3.   Bake until the carrots soften and begin to brown, about 40 minutes, flipping after about 20 minutes.

Nutrition:

- Calories: 142
- Fats: 7 g
- Sodium: 322 mg
- Carbs: 22 g
- Fiber: 1 g
- Protein: 1 g

21.   No-Fat Biscuits

Preparation Time: 10 minutes

Cooking Time: 25 minutes

Servings: 6

Ingredients:

- Nonstick cooking spray

- 2 cups all-purpose flour

- ¾ tsp. baking soda

- 2 tsp. baking powder

- A pinch sea salt

- 1 ¼ cups nonfat plain yogurt

Directions:

1. Preheat the oven to 425°F. Spray a rimmed baking sheet with nonstick cooking spray.

2. In a medium bowl, whisk together the flour, baking soda, baking powder, and salt.

3. Fold in the yogurt until just mixed.

4. Use a large spoon to form 6 biscuits on the prepared baking sheet.

5. Bake until the biscuits are golden brown, about 20 to 25 minutes.

Nutrition:

- Calories: 161

- Fats: 0 g

- Sodium: 373 mg

- Carbs: 34 g

- Fiber: 1 g

- Protein: 7 g

22.   Easy Cornbread

Preparation Time: 20 minutes

Cooking Time: 20 minutes

Servings: 6

Ingredients:

- Nonstick cooking spray

- ¾ cup all-purpose flour

- 1 ½ cups cornmeal

- 1 tbsp. baking powder

- ¼ tsp. sea salt

- 1 large egg, beaten

- 1 cup nonfat milk

Directions:

1.   Preheat the oven to 425°F. Spray a 9-inch baking pan with nonstick cooking spray.

2.   In a medium bowl, whisk together the flour, cornmeal, baking powder, and salt.

3.   In a small bowl, whisk together the egg and milk.

4.   Add the wet ingredients to the dry ingredients and fold together until just combined. Pour into the prepared pan.

5.   Bake until browned, about 20 minutes.

Nutrition:

- Calories: 188

- Fats: 2 g

- Sodium: 380 mg

- Carbs: 37 g

- Fiber: 3 g

- Protein: 6 g

23.   Shredded Brussels Sprouts

Preparation Time: 10 minutes

Cooking Time: 7 minutes

Servings: 4

Ingredients:

- 1 tbsp. olive oil

- 8 ounces Brussels sprouts, shredded or julienned

- ½ tsp. sea salt

Directions:

1.   Place a large nonstick skillet over medium-high heat and add the olive oil. Once the oil is shimmering, add the Brussels sprouts and salt. Cook, stirring occasionally until the sprouts are browned, about 5 to 7 minutes.

Nutrition:

*   Calories: 54

*   Fats: 4 g

*   Sodium: 305 mg

*   Carbs: 5 g

*   Fiber: 2 g

*   Protein: 2 g

24.   Maple-Ginger Roasted Beets

Preparation Time: 10 minutes

Cooking Time: 1 hour

Servings: 4

Ingredients:

*   8 oz. beets, peeled and quartered

*   2 tbsp. olive oil

*   ½ tsp. sea salt

*   1 tbsp. fresh ginger, grated

- ¼ cup pure maple syrup

Directions:

1.   Preheat the oven to 400°F.

2.   Place the beets on a rimmed baking sheet and drizzle with the olive oil. Toss to coat. Sprinkle with the salt and ginger.

3.   Roast for 30 minutes. Remove from the oven. Drizzle the beets with the syrup and stir to mix. Return to the oven and continue roasting for 30 minutes more.

Nutrition:

- Calories: 137

- Fats: 7 g

- Sodium: 337 mg

- Carbs: 19 g

- Fiber: 2 g

- Protein: 1 g

25.   Ginger-Cumin Kale Chips

Preparation Time: 10 minutes

Cooking Time: 20 minutes

Servings: 6

Ingredients:

•   1 bunch kale, stems removed and leaves trimmed

•   1 tbsp. olive oil

•   ½ tsp. sea salt

•   1 tbsp. fresh ginger, grated

•   ½ tsp. ground cumin

Directions:

1.   Preheat the oven to 350°F. Line a rimmed baking sheet with parchment paper.

2.   In a large bowl, toss the kale leaves with the olive oil, salt, ginger, and cumin.

3.   Spread in an even layer on the prepared baking pan.

4.   Bake until the kale is crisp and starting to brown, about 20 minutes, flipping after about 10 minutes.

Nutrition:

•   Calories: 40

•   Fats: 3 g

•   Sodium: 209 mg

•   Carbs: 4 g

•   Fiber: 1 g

- Protein: 1 g

26.   Ginger Mashed Sweet Potatoes

Preparation Time: 10 minutes

Cooking Time: 15 minutes

Servings: 4

Ingredients:

- 2 sweet potatoes, peeled and cut into 1-inch pieces

- 2 cups water

- 1 tbsp. fresh ginger, grated

- ½ cup nonfat milk or nondairy milk

- ¼ cup nonfat plain yogurt

- ½ tsp. sea salt

Directions:

1.   Place the sweet potatoes in a large pot and cover with at least 2 inches of water. Place over medium-high heat and bring to a boil.

2.   Cover and cook until the potatoes are tender, about 15 minutes.

3.   Drain the potatoes and return them to the pot. Add the ginger, milk, yogurt, and salt.

4.   Mash with a potato masher until smooth, and then stir well to combine.

Nutrition:

- Calories: 87
- Fats: <1 g
- Sodium: 322 mg
- Carbs: 19 g
- Fiber: 2 g
- Protein: 3 g

27.   Calm Carrot Salad

Preparation Time: 10 minutes

Cooking Time: 0 minutes

Servings: 2

Ingredients:

- 2 tbsp. Splenda®
- 2 tbsp. raisins
- 2 tsp. olive oil
- ¼ tsp. salt
- ¼ lb. mesclun greens
- 1 lb. carrots, trimmed and grated

- 1 tsp. dried oregano

Directions:

1. Mix oregano, Splenda®, salt, raisins, and olive oil in a medium bowl.

2. Toss in the carrots and mix well to coat.

3. Adjust the seasoning with salt.

4. Serve over the mesclun greens.

Nutrition:

- Calories: 144
- Fats: 0.4 g
- Carbs: 8 g
- Protein: 5.6 g

28. Millet Cauliflower Mash

Preparation Time: 10 minutes

Cooking Time: 30 minutes

Servings: 4

Ingredients:

- 1 tsp. tamari
- 3 cups water
- 1 cup cauliflower florets

- 2 tsp. parsley sprig

- 1 cup millet

- ¼ tsp. salt

Directions:

1. Roast the millet in a nonstick pan for 5 minutes.

2. Boil the water in a large pan on high heat, then add the cauliflower, salt, and millet.

3. Cover the dish with the lid, then cook for 25 minutes on low heat.

4. Stir in the tamari and cook for 5 minutes.

5. Lightly mash the cauliflower mixture.

6. Garnish with parsley and serve.

Nutrition:

- Calories: 454

- Fats: 4 g

- Carbs: 30 g

- Protein: 4 g

29. Spinach and Dill Dip

Preparation Time: 5 minutes

Cooking Time: 3 minutes

Servings: 4

Ingredients:

- 2 cups baby spinach

- ½ tsp. lemon zest, grated

- ¼ tsp. sea salt

- 1 cup lactose-free nonfat plain yogurt

- 2 tbsp. fresh dill, chopped

Directions:

1.	In a large nonstick skillet, add the spinach, lemon zest, and sea salt. Cook, stirring, until the spinach wilts, 2 to 3 minutes. Remove from the heat and allow the spinach to cool.

2.	In a small bowl, combine the cooled spinach, yogurt, and dill, stirring to combine.

3.	Serve.

Nutrition:

- Calories: 68

- Protein: 4 g

- Fats: 4 g

- Carbs: 5 g

30.	Zucchini Hummus

Preparation Time: 5 minutes

Cooking Time: 0 minutes

Servings: 4

Ingredients:

- 1 medium zucchini, chopped
- 1 tbsp. olive oil
- 1 tbsp. tahini
- 1 tsp. fresh dill, chopped
- ½ tsp. lemon zest, grated
- ½ tsp. sea salt

Directions:

1. In a blender or food processor, combine all the ingredients. Blend until smooth. Serve.

Nutrition:

- Calories: 60
- Protein: 6 g
- Fats: 3 g
- Carbs: 2 g

31. Zucchini and Salmon Canapés

Preparation Time: 15 minutes

Cooking Time: 0 minutes

Servings: 4

Ingredients:

- 4 oz. canned salmon, drained, rinsed, and flaked
- ¼ cup lactose-free nonfat plain yogurt
- 1 tsp. orange zest, grated
- 1 tsp. fresh tarragon, chopped
- ½ tsp. sea salt
- 1 zucchini, cut into 12 rounds

Directions:

1. In a small bowl, combine the salmon, yogurt, orange zest, tarragon, and salt.
2. Spoon onto the zucchini rounds.
3. Serve.

Nutrition:

- Calories: 53
- Protein: 7 g
- Fats: 2 g
- Carbs: 1 g

32.   Olive Tapenade

Preparation Time: 15 minutes

Cooking Time: 0 minutes

Servings: 4

Ingredients:

- ½ cup black olives, pitted and chopped
- ½ anchovy fillet, chopped
- 1 tbsp. olive oil
- 2 tbsp. fresh basil, chopped
- ½ tsp. lemon zest

Directions:

1.   In a small bowl, mix all the ingredients until well combined.

2.   Serve.

Nutrition:

- Calories: 51
- Protein: 0 g
- Fats: 5 g
- Carbs: 1 g

33.   Sweet Potato French Fries

Preparation Time: 10 minutes

Cooking Time: 20 minutes

Servings: 2

Ingredients:

- 1 sweet potato, peeled and cut into ¼-inch matchsticks

- 1 tsp. ground cumin

- ½ tsp. sea salt

- 1 tbsp. olive oil

Directions:

1.   Preheat the oven to 450°F.

2.   In a bowl, toss together the sweet potato sticks, cumin, salt, and olive oil.

3.   Spread in a single layer on a rimmed baking sheet.

4.   Bake, turning once with a spatula until the fries are browned and tender, about 20 minutes. Serve.

Nutrition:

- Calories: 115

- Protein: 1 g

- Fats: 7 g

- Carbs: 14 g

34.	Chicken Fajita Salad

Preparation Time: 10 minutes

Cooking Time: 5 minutes

Servings: 4

Ingredients:

For the Marinade/Dressing:

- 3 tbsp. olive oil

- 2 tbsp. cilantro, chopped

- 2 cloves garlic, crushed

- 1 tsp. Splenda®

- ¾ tsp. red chili flakes

- ½ tsp. ground Cumin

- 1 tsp. salt

For the Salad:

- 4 chicken thigh fillets, skin removed

- ½ yellow bell pepper, sliced and deseeded

- ½ red bell pepper, deseeded and sliced

- ½ an onion, sliced

- 5 cups Romaine, (or cos) lettuce leaves, washed and dried

- 2 avocados, sliced

- Extra cilantro leaves to garnish

- Sour cream, (optional) to serve

Directions:

1. To make the marinade combine all of its ingredients in a bowl.

2. Season the chicken pieces with this marinade.

3. Marinate the meat in the refrigerator for 2 hours.

4. Heat 1 teaspoon of oil in a grill pan. Sear the chicken from sides until golden brown.

5. Transfer the chicken to a plate.

6. Sauté the onions and the pepper in the same pan.

7. Slice the chicken and toss it with the pepper, onion, avocado, and leaves in a bowl.

8. Stir in the salad dressing.

9. Toss well and serve.

Nutrition:

- Calories: 184

- Fats: 37 g

- Saturated Fat: 8 g

- Cholesterol: 110 mg

- Sodium: 689 mg

- Carbs: 13 g

- Fiber: 8 g

- Sugar: 3 g

- Protein 19 g

35.   Playgroup Granola Bars

Preparation Time: 10 minutes

Cooking Time: 35 minutes

Servings: 4

Ingredients:

- 2 cups rolled oats

- ¾ cup packed coconut sugar

- ½ cup wheat germ

- ¾ tsp. ground cinnamon

- 1 cup almond flour

- ¾ cup raisins (optional)

- ¾ tsp. salt

- ½ cup honey
- 1 egg, beaten
- ½ cup vegetable oil
- 2 tsp. vanilla extract

Directions:

1. Set the oven at 350ºF to preheat. Grease a 9x13-inch pan with cooking spray.

2. Toss the oats with the wheat germ, flour, raisins, salt, cinnamon, and coconut sugar in a bowl

3. Add the egg white, oil, vanilla, and honey to the mixture.

4. Mix well with your hands and then transfer it to the baking pan.

5. Bake for 35 minutes, or until golden brown around the edges.

6. Slice and serve.

Nutrition:

- Calories: 307
- Fats: 25 g
- Saturated Fat: 5 g
- Cholesterol: 16 mg
- Sodium: 372 mg

- Carbs: 16 g
- Fiber: 5 g
- Sugar: 4 g
- Protein: 10 g

1.   Seafood Paella Recipe

Preparation Time: 10 minutes

Cooking Time: 22 minutes

Servings: 4

Ingredients:

- 1 ½-pint fish stock

- A pinch saffron

- 1 ½ tbsp. extra-virgin olive oil

- 1 large onion, finely chopped

- 3 garlic cloves, crushed

- 1 (1 ¼-oz.) pack, flat-leaf parsley, leaves chopped

- 1 tsp. black pepper

- 2 ¼ cups (8-oz.) Spanish paella rice

- 1 cup red bell pepper, chopped

- 2 ¼ cup jars roasted peppers, drain and rinse them

- 1 ⅓ cup (6-oz.) raw black tiger prawns

- 1 ¼ cup (5-oz.) live mussels, cleaned and debearded

- 1 ¼ cup raw squid rings
- 1 lemon, cut into wedges

Directions:

1.   Boil the fish stock with saffron and keep it aside.

2.   Preheat the oil to sauté the onion for 5 minutes.

3.   Add the garlic, bell pepper, parsley, and black pepper. Stir-cook for 2 minutes.

4.   Stir in the rice and stock, and cook for 10 minutes.

5.   Add in roasted peppers and cook for 5 minutes.

6.   Place prawns, mussels, and squid rings in the pan.

7.   Cook for 5 minutes, then take off the heat.

8.   Cover the pan with foil and let it sit for 5 minutes.

9.   Garnish with the parsley.

10.   SERVE.

Nutrition:

- Calories: 272
- Fats: 11 g

- Saturated Fat: 3 g
- Cholesterol: 66 mg
- Sodium: 288 mg
- Carbs: 10 g
- Fiber: 4 g
- Sugar: 0 g
- Protein: 33 g

2.   Sicilian Seafood Stew

Preparation Time: 10 minutes

Cooking Time: 20 minutes

Servings: 4

Ingredients:

- 2 tbsp. olive oil
- 1 onion, chopped
- 2 sticks celery, chopped
- 2 garlic cloves, chopped, plus an extra clove
- 1 anchovy, rinsed
- 1 tsp. dried chili flakes
- 1 cup red bell pepper

- ½ cup nonfat yogurt

- 2 cups vegetable stock

- 3 cups raw peeled prawns

- 2 cups new potatoes

- 1 lemon, zested and juiced

- 1 tsp. baby capers

- 1 tsp. flat-leaf parsley, chopped

Directions:

1.	Preheat the olive oil in a suitable pot, and sauté the celery, onion, anchovy, garlic, and chili.

2.	Season with pepper and salt. Stir-cook for 5 minutes.

3.	Meanwhile, boil the potatoes until al dente. Cut them into thick slices.

4.	Add the stock, yogurt, and bell pepper to the pan, and cook for 15 minutes.

5.	Place the prawns in the pan along with the potatoes, capers, lemon zest, and juice.

6.	Cook for 5 minutes and then serve.

Nutrition:

- Calories: 557

- Fats: 29 g

- Saturated Fat: 22 g

- Cholesterol: 550 mg

- Sodium: 1800 mg

- Carbs: 25 g

- Fiber: 3 g

- Sugar: 0.3 g

- Protein: 47 g

3.   Seafood Stew

Preparation Time: 5 minutes

Cooking Time: 17 minutes

Servings: 4

Ingredients:

- 1 large onion, finely sliced

- 1 garlic clove, finely chopped

- Black pepper, to taste

- 1 cup nonfat yogurt

- 2 cups chicken stock

- 4 ¼ cups skinless white fish fillets, chopped into large chunks

- 1 ⅓ cups raw peeled king prawns

- 2 cups mussels, cleaned and debearded

• A small bunch flat-leaf parsley leaves, roughly chopped

• Crusty bread and almond butter, to serve (optional)

Directions:

1. Preheat the oil in a pan and sauté for onions for 5 minutes.

2. Add the pepper and garlic, and stir-cook for 2 minutes.

3. Pour in the stock and yogurt. Cook for 10 minutes.

4. Place the fish chunks in the pan and cook for 2 minutes.

5. Stir in the mussels and prawns. Cover the pan and cook for 3 minutes.

6. Garnish with parsley.

7. Serve.

Nutrition:

• Calories: 301

• Fats: 12.2 g

• Saturated Fat: 2.4 g

• Cholesterol: 110 mg

• Sodium: 276 mg

- Carbs: 5 g
- Fiber: 0.9 g
- Sugar: 1.4 g
- Protein: 28.8 g

4.   Fritto Misto With Gremolata

Preparation Time: 5 minutes

Cooking Time: 15 minutes

Servings: 4

Ingredients:

For the Gremolata:

- A small bunch flat-leaf parsley, finely chopped
- 1 lemon, zested
- ½ tsp. garlic, finely chopped

For the Fritto Misto:

- ⅓ cup (3-oz.) almond flour
- ¼ tsp. black pepper
- 2 ¼ cups cod fillet, bones removed and cut into bite-sized pieces
- 1 ⅓ cups mixed seafood

- 6 tbsp. olive oil

- Good-quality mayo, to serve

Directions:

1.   Mix all the ingredients for the gremolata.

2.   Combine the flour with the black pepper and seasoning in a bowl.

3.   Dip the seafood in the flour mixture.

4.   Preheat the oil in a frying pan and fry the coated seafood until golden brown.

5.   Serve.

Nutrition:

- Calories: 310

- Fats: 2.4 g

- Saturated Fat: 0.1 g

- Cholesterol: 320 mg

- Sodium: 350 mg

- Carbs: 12.2 g

- Fiber: 0.7 g

- Sugar: 0.7 g

- Protein: 44.3 g

5.   Fritto Misto

Preparation Time: 5 minutes

Cooking Time: 10 minutes

Servings: 2

Ingredients:

- 1 cup Vegetable oil for deep frying

- 1 egg

- ½ pint whole milk

- 1 lb. mixed raw seafood, cut into pieces

- 1 zucchini, cut into batons

- ⅔ cup (4-oz.) almond flour

- 6 tbsp. corn flour

- ⅔ cup (4-oz.) semolina

Directions:

1.   Preheat the oil to 320ºF in a deep pan.

2.   Beat the milk with the egg white and seasonings.

3.   Add the seafood and zucchini to the milk.

4.   Combine corn flour, semolina, and flour in a bowl.

5.   Dip the seafood and zucchini in the flour mixture, and shake off the excess.

6.   Add the oil to a deep pan and heat to fry until golden.

7.   Serve.

Nutrition:

- Calories: 372
- Fats: 1.1 g
- Saturated Fat: 3.8 g
- Cholesterol: 10 mg
- Sodium: 749 mg
- Carbs: 4.9 g
- Fiber: 0.2 g
- Sugar: 0.2 g
- Protein: 33.5 g

6.   Fish Soup

Preparation Time: 5 minutes

Cooking Time: 1 hour

Servings: 2

Ingredients:

- 2 tsp Olive oil
- 2 small onions, finely chopped

- 2 carrots, finely chopped

- 2 celery stalks, finely chopped

- 4 garlic cloves, finely chopped

- 1–2 sweet peppers, deseeded and finely chopped

- 2 ½ pints vegetable stock

- 4 cups fish stock

- 2 anchovy fillets in oil, drained

- Salt, pepper

- Pepper, pepper

- 2 ¼ cups (8-oz.) monkfish tail, all bones removed and flesh cut into cubes

- 2 ¼ cups (8-oz.) frozen seafood, defrosted and rinsed

- 2 handfuls small soup pasta

- A handful olives (black or green), pitted and finely chopped

- Fresh crusty bread, to serve

Directions:

1.   Preheat the olive oil in the pan and sauté the onions, celery, peppers, and garlic until golden.

2.   Stir in the stock, anchovy, and pepper.

162

3.   Cover the lid and cook for 40 minutes.

4.   Stir in the monkfish tail, pasta, and seafood.

5.   Cover and cook for 20 minutes.

6.   Serve with olives on top.

7.   Enjoy.

Nutrition:

*   Calories: 581

*   Fats: 23 g

*   Saturated Fat: 4 g

*   Cholesterol: 49 mg

*   Sodium: 257 mg

*   Carbs: 3.6 g

*   Fiber: 10 g

*   Sugar: 0.5 g

*   Protein: 58 g

7.   Chicken Chasseur

Preparation Time: 5 minutes

Cooking Time: 30 minutes

Servings: 4

Ingredients:

- 4 chicken legs
- 1 tbsp. olive oil
- 1 onion, finely sliced
- 2 garlic cloves, finely sliced
- 2 ¼ cups (8-oz.) chestnut mushrooms, cut into 4 if small and 6 if large
- 3 ½ cups chicken stock
- 1 bay leaf
- 1 thyme sprig
- 1 cup nonfat yogurt
- 1 red bell pepper, chopped
- A small handful of tarragon, chopped
- Mashed potatoes, to serve

Directions:

1.	Sear the chicken legs in some oil until golden brown.

2.	Remove the chicken and sauté onion until soft.

3.	Add mushrooms and garlic until golden.

4.	Stir in nonfat yogurt, bay leaf, thyme, red bell pepper, and chicken stock.

5.   Boil the mixture and then reduce it to a simmer. Add the chicken legs.

6.   Cook for 30 minutes and add the tarragon.

7.   Serve.

Nutrition:

- Calories: 529

- Fats: 17 g

- Saturated Fat: 3 g

- Cholesterol: 65 mg

- Sodium: 391 mg

- Carbs: 55 g

- Fiber: 6 g

- Sugar: 8 g

- Protein: 41 g

8.   Smoky Chicken Traybake

Preparation Time: 10 minutes

Cooking Time: 45 minutes

Servings: 4

Ingredients:

- 1 (2-lb.) pack chicken thighs and drumsticks

- Olive oil, for greasing

- 1 red bell pepper, deseeded and roughly chopped

- 2 yellow bell peppers, deseeded and roughly chopped

- 2 red onions, peeled and sliced into wedges

- ½ cups barbecue sauce

- 7 ¼ cups sweet potatoes, scrubbed and cut into wedges

- ⅔ cup sour cream

- Coriander leaves, to garnish

- Guacamole, to serve

Directions:

1. Set the oven to 400ºF. Score the skin of the thighs.

2. Place them with the peppers and the red onion in the roasting pan.

3. Mix all the remaining ingredients.

4. Top the chicken and vegetables with this paste.

5.   Roast the chicken for 15 minutes and then add sweet potato.

6.   Turn all the drumsticks and bake for 30 minutes.

7.   Serve.

Nutrition:

- Calories: 284

- Fats: 25 g

- Saturated Fat: 1 g

- Cholesterol: 49 mg

- Sodium: 460 mg

- Carbs: 35 g

- Fiber: 2 g

- Sugar: 6 g

- Protein: 26 g

9.   Chicken and Orzo Bake

Preparation Time: 5 minutes

Cooking Time: 40 minutes

Servings: 4

Ingredients:

- ½ tbsp. olive oil

- 4 (2 1/5-lb.) pack bone-in chicken thighs
- 2 onions, finely chopped
- 2 celery sticks, finely chopped
- 1 carrot, peeled and finely chopped
- 1 garlic clove, finely chopped
- 1 tsp. fennel seeds
- 2 cups orzo
- 1 chicken stock cube, made up with 2 cups hot water
- 2 cups frozen broccoli florets
- A handful fresh dill, chopped
- 1 lemon, cut into wedges to serve
- Pepper, to taste

Directions:

1. Preheat the oil in a deep cooking pan.

2. Season the chicken and cook for 5 minutes per side.

3. Remove the chicken from the cooking pan and keep it aside.

4. Drain the excess fat and keep it aside.

5. Add the onion, carrot, celery, garlic, and fennel seeds to the pan.

6.   Stir-cook for 10 minutes and then add stock and orzo.

7.   Return the chicken to the pan.

8.   Boil the mixture and cook on simmer for 5 minutes.

9.   Add the broccoli and cook for 20 minutes.

10.   GARNISH WITH DILL AND PEPPER.

11.   SERVE.

Nutrition:

- Calories: 152

- Fats: 4 g

- Saturated Fat: 2 g

- Cholesterol: 65 mg

- Sodium: 220 mg

- Carbs: 1 tsp.

- Fiber: 0 g

- Sugar: 1 g

- Protein: 26 g

10.   One-Pot Roast

Preparation Time: 10 minutes

Cooking Time: 50 minutes

Servings: 8

Ingredients:

- 8 chicken thighs
- 1 ½ lb. sweet potato, cut into chunks
- 2 cups (7-oz.) chorizo sausage, sliced
- 1 bulb garlic, broken into cloves
- 2 tbsp. grapeseed oil
- ⅓ cup chicken stock
- 1 lemon, halved
- 2 zucchinis, cut into thick batons
- 1 red chili, deseeded and sliced
- 2 1/6 cup (8-oz.) baby spinach
- 2 tbsp. parsley, chopped
- A pinch salt
- A pinch black pepper

Directions:

1.   Set the oven to 400ºF.

2.   Place the chicken with the sweet potato in a roasting pan.

3.   Top the chicken with garlic, grapeseed oil, stock, and lemon juice.

4.   Bake for 50 minutes. Add the zucchini, chili, and chorizo after 30 minutes of baking.

5.   Garnish with the parsley and spinach.

6.   Serve.

Nutrition:

- Calories: 188

- Fats: 8 g

- Saturated Fat: 1 g

- Cholesterol: 0 mg

- Sodium: 339 mg

- Carbs: 8 g

- Fiber: 1 g

- Sugar: 2 g

- Protein: 13 g

11.   Beef Curry

Preparation Time: 10 minutes

Cooking Time: 22 minutes

Servings: 4

Ingredients:

- 14 oz. beef rump, sliced thinly
- ¼ cup sunflower oil
- 1 cup brown rice
- 4 ¼ cups boiling water
- 1 tbsp. fresh ginger, minced
- A few slices of fresh ginger
- 2 garlic cloves, minced
- 1 tsp. ground cumin
- 1 tsp. ground coriander
- 1 tsp. turmeric
- 1 tsp. ground black pepper
- ½ tsp. chili powder
- ½ tsp. ground ginger
- ½ cup frozen peas
- Coriander sprigs, to garnish
- Salt, to taste

Directions:

1. Boil the rice in salted water and cook for 12 minutes. Drain and keep aside.

172

2.   Preheat the sunflower oil in the pan, and sear the beef until brown.

3.   Remove the beef to the plate lined with a paper towel.

4.   Add the ginger and garlic, and sauté for few minutes.

5.   Stir in the spices and water.

6.   Cook for 10 minutes, then add peas.

7.   Adjust the seasoning, and garnish with coriander.

8.   Serve.

Nutrition:

- Calories: 301
- Fats: 15.8 g
- Saturated Fat: 2.7 g
- Cholesterol: 75 mg
- Sodium: 1189 mg
- Carbs: 11.7 g
- Fiber: 0.3 g
- Sugar: 0.1 g
- Protein: 28.2 g

12.   Beef Schnitzel

Preparation Time: 10 minutes

Cooking Time: 30 minutes

Servings: 6

Ingredients:

- 4 tbsp. almond flour
- 1 large egg, beaten
- 1 ¼ cup (5-oz.) breadcrumbs
- 2 (3 1/6) cups beef medallion steaks
- 2 tbsp. olive oil
- 1 lemon, cut into wedges to serve

For the slaw:

- 2 raw beetroots, peeled and grated
- 1 large carrot, peeled and grated
- ½ red onion, peeled and finely sliced
- 2 stalks celery, finely sliced
- ½ pack dill, leaves chopped
- 1 lemon, zested and juiced
- 1 tbsp. extra-virgin olive oil

Directions:

1.	Combine everything for the slaw in a bowl. Adjust the seasoning with salt.

2.	Mix the flour with the lemon zest and salt.

3.	Beat the egg white in a bowl, and spread breadcrumbs in a shallow bowl.

4.	Place each beef medallion in between 2 sheets of parchment paper.

5.	Pound the meat using a rolling pin to reduce the thickness.

6.	First, dip the meat into the flour mixture; then add the egg, and then breadcrumbs.

7.	Preheat the oil in a frying pan, and cook the coated meat for 2 minutes per side.

8.	Serve with slaw.

Nutrition:

•	Calories: 308

•	Fats: 20.5 g

•	Saturated Fat: 3 g

•	Cholesterol: 0 mg

•	Sodium: 688 mg

•	Carbs: 10.3 g

•	Sugar: 1.4 g

•	Fiber: 4.3 g

- Protein: 49 g

13.   Beef Massaman Curry

Preparation Time: 10 minutes

Cooking Time: 31 minutes

Servings: 6

Ingredients:

- 1 ½ tbsp. vegetable oil

- 2 onions, chopped

- 2 ¼ cups Thai jasmine rice

- 2 cups Thai massaman paste

- 3 cups potatoes, cut into 2 cm-thick slices

- 5 ¼ cups cooked roast beef, cut into chunks

- 1 ⅓ cups pack baby corn and snap peas

- Water, as needed

- 2 tbsp Star anise

Directions:

1.   Preheat the oil in a deep-frying pan, and sauté the onions for 10 minutes on low heat.

2.   Boil the rice in salted water for 10 minutes, and then drain and keep them aside.

3.   Add the massaman paste and cook for 1 minute.

4.   Put in the sliced potato, coconut milk, and star anise.

5.   Cook this mixture for 15 minutes.

6.   Add snap peas, a splash of water, corn, and beef.

7.   Cook for 5 minutes, then serve.

Nutrition:

- Calories: 231

- Fats: 20.1 g

- Saturated Fat: 2.4 g

- Cholesterol: 110 mg

- Sodium: 941 mg

- Carbs: 20.1 g

- Fiber: 0.9 g

- Sugar: 1.4 g

- Protein: 14.6 g

14.   Barbecued Rump of Beef in Dijon

Preparation Time: 10 minutes

Cooking Time: 1 hour and 45 minutes

Servings: 4

Ingredients:

- 2 lb. beef top rump joint
- 2 tbsp. fresh tarragon, roughly chopped
- 2 tsp. black pepper
- 1 tbsp. Dijon mustard
- 2 tbsp. olive oil

Directions:

1. Keep the meat in a shallow dish and toss with tarragon, mustard, oil, and pepper to season.

2. Marinate the meat in the refrigerator for 1 ½ hours.

3. Preheat the grill and grill for 15 minutes.

4. Carve and serve.

Nutrition:

- Calories: 280
- Fats: 3.5 g
- Saturated Fat: 0.1 g
- Cholesterol: 320 mg
- Sodium: 350 mg
- Carbs: 7.6 g

- Fiber: 0.7 g

- Sugar: 0.7 g

- Protein: 11.2 g

15.   Roast Rib of Beef

Preparation Time: 10 minutes

Cooking Time: 45 minutes

Servings: 6

Ingredients:

- 2 Knorr® Beef Stock Cubes

- 1 tbsp. olive oil

- 3 lb. rib of beef

- 5 small leeks

- 6 parsnips, peeled and halved

- 6 carrots, peeled and halved

- 4 shallots, peeled and halved

- Celery sticks, cut into large chunks, for serving

- Fresh sage leaves, for serving

Directions:

1.   Set the oven to 400ºF.

2.   Mix 1 Knorr beef cube with 1 tablespoon of oil and rub this paste onto the beef.

3.   Sear the beef in a greased pan until brown, then transfer them to a roasting pan.

4.   Sauté the leeks in the same pan until golden, and place them around the beef.

5.   Now sauté carrots and parsnips in the pan and also transfer them to the roasting pan.

6.   Top the beef with sage, celery, and shallots.

7.   Bake for 45 minutes.

8.   Serve.

Nutrition:

- Calories: 472

- Fats: 11.1 g

- Saturated Fat: 5.8 g

- Cholesterol: 610 mg

- Sodium: 749 mg

- Carbs: 19.9 g

- Fiber: 0.2 g

- Sugar: 0.2 g

- Protein: 13.5 g

16.   Beef Wellington with Stilton

Preparation Time: 5 minutes

Cooking Time: 55 minutes

Servings: 4

Ingredients:

- 2 tbsp. olive oil
- 2 tbsp. pine nuts
- 1 garlic clove, crushed
- 4 tbsp. horseradish sauce
- ¼ cup (2-oz.) mature stilton, crumbled
- 1 oz. fresh white breadcrumbs
- 1 (1 ½-lb.) beef fillet piece
- 3 ⅓ cups (13-oz.) ready-rolled puff pastry
- Beaten egg, to glaze

Directions:

1.   Preheat 1 tablespoon of oil in a frying pan and sauté the pine nuts for 1 minute.

2.   Toss in the garlic and set the mixture aside to cool.

3.　　Combine the stilton, horseradish, breadcrumbs, black pepper, and pine nuts mixture.

4.　　Heat more oil in a pan and sear beef fillet for 3 minutes per side, or until brown.

5.　　Adjust the oven to 400ºF.

6.　　Top the beef with the horseradish mixture.

7.　　Spread the pastry sheet and top the beef pan with it.

8.　　Brush the pastry with the beaten egg white.

9.　　Seal the edges and bake for 40 minutes.

10.　　SERVE.

Nutrition:

- Calories: 327

- Fats: 3.5 g

- Saturated Fat: 0.5 g

- Cholesterol: 162 mg

- Sodium: 142 mg

- Carbs: 33.6 g

- Fiber: 0.4 g

- Sugar: 0.5 g

- Protein: 24.5 g

17.   Marinated Lamb Steaks

Preparation Time: 10 minutes

Cooking Time: 30 minutes

Servings: 6

Ingredients:

- 6 lamb leg steaks
- ½ cup dark coconut aminos
- 1 tbsp. curry powder
- 1 tsp. ground ginger
- 1 tbsp. nonfat yogurt
- 1 tbsp. olive oil
- Salt, to taste
- Pepper, to taste
- 2 cups fresh potatoes
- ⅔ cup pot natural yogurt
- A bunch mint
- A bunch spring onions
- Salted water, as needed

Directions:

1.   Combine everything for the marinade and rub it over the lamb steaks.

2.   Let it marinate for 1 hour at room temperature.

3.   Meanwhile, boil the potatoes in the salted water, drain them, and let them cool down.

4.   Mix the yogurt with spring onion and mint.

5.   Toss in the potatoes and seasonings.

6.   Preheat the grill and grill the lamb steaks for 3 minutes per side.

7.   Serve with the potato mixture.